MW00986315

SWEET SURRENDER

BREAKING STRONGHOLDS

TERESA SHIELDS PARKER

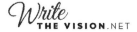

SWEET SURRENDER
BREAKING STRONGHOLDS

Printed in the USA

ISBN: 978-0-9861592-4-4

Published by Write the Vision | Columbia, Missouri

Write
THE VISION.NET

CONTACT THE AUTHOR AT
www.teresashieldsparker.com

*"For though we live in the
world, we do not wage
war as the world does.
The weapons we fight with are
not the weapons of the world.
On the contrary, they have divine
power to demolish strongholds.
We demolish arguments and
every pretension that sets itself up
against the knowledge of God,
and we take captive every thought
to make it obedient to Christ."*

2 CORINTHIANS 10:3-5 NIV

DEDICATION

To Russ Hardesty:

My life is richer and fuller because of how you
challenge me to always reach higher.
Before I met you, I was a broken, unhealthy, sad blob.
Now I am a whole, healthy, happy woman.
I finally know what it means to live
in overflowing abundance.
Thank you for what you do and who you are.

"Don't copy the behavior and customs of this world, but let God transform you into a new person by changing the way you think. Then you will learn to know God's will for you, which is good and pleasing and perfect."

ROMANS 12:2 NLT

ACKNOWLEDGEMENTS

There are people without whom this book would have not been possible. First, huge applause goes to Wendy Walters for the cover design, formatting work, foreword and ongoing moral support throughout this process. It would be extremely difficult for me to publish a book without Wendy.

A big shout out goes to the special people who helped read, give feedback and proofread the book: Marilyn Logan, Linda Ordway, Candy Hamilton and others. Thanks to the behind-the-scenes prayer intercessors who have prayed me through all six books in the Sweet Series. I value each of you beyond words. You kept me sane and on track when it felt like I couldn't go on. There were many days like that. I felt your prayers. They buoyed me up.

Thanks to my children, Andrew Parker and Jenny Church, for always being there to help in any way I ask. Thanks also to my sister, Renee Shields Allen, and my brother, Mark Randall Shields, for their ongoing support of whatever I choose to reveal from our childhoods.

One last big thank you goes to my sweet husband who puts up with my late nights and incessant talk about whatever book I'm writing. I love you to the moon and back again, Roy Parker. God gave me the best gift ever when He gave me you.

Sweet Grace for Your Journey,

Teresa

C O N T E N T S

F O R E W O R D

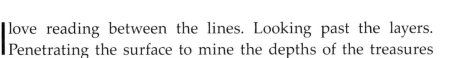

I love reading between the lines. Looking past the layers. Penetrating the surface to mine the depths of the treasures which lie beneath our view.

In 2013, I hosted my first Release the Writer conference at a property in Missouri. I do a few each year now, and each is special to me for different reasons, but that first one is deeply embedded in my memory as being very special.

At the time, my daughter was my assistant, and she was handling event registration. A woman walked in with a check in hand and plunked it down on the table matter-of-factly. She was a journalist. Educated. Experienced. She was there against her will at the arm-twisting of the friend who owned the venue we had chosen to host our event. Though she was not rude, she did not smile. The woman indicated that she was not sure we would be offering anything at this seminar she did not already know.

Kate handed her the workbook and registration packet, and she made her way inside, ignoring all the chairs set up classroom style behind tables, and picked a spot off in the corner by herself. I leaned in to Kate and said, "Better not deposit that check; I have a feeling we may need to give it back before the day ends!"

That inaugural Release the Writer was a five-day event, and we went through the material, allowing the Holy Spirit to infuse it with prophetic destiny, hope, the rekindling of dreams, and the joy of Jesus. The woman warmed up considerably, gradually dropped her guard, entered the discussions and freely gave herself to the exercises. Not only did we not need to refund her, but she also signed up for a private one-on-one coaching session at the event's conclusion.

That woman was Teresa Shields Parker—and you now hold the sixth book she has published since attending Release the Writer in 2013. That shy, dry, make-it-through-life-as-best-as-you-can woman has blossomed into a force to be reckoned with! She has coached hundreds of people through her Christian weight loss programs, walking them through inner healing and freedom. She has been on major television and radio shows, national broadcasters have picked up her blogs and podcast, and she is a social media influencer. She now wears colorful clothes and even makeup. She smiles often and is dedicated to helping others break the strongholds that keep them from living fully alive and free in the purpose for which they were created.

She's a better writer than I will ever be—a gifted storyteller with the ability to connect emotionally with her audience and bring home truths without banging you over the head with them. You'll enjoy this book. You will likely find yourself between the pages and recognize issues you grapple with and challenges you face.

In those moments, it is there where Teresa will meet you and offer you her hand to guide you along the way. It's a ditch she's been in and knows the way out. It's a place she vividly remembers with enough acrimony to be passionate about helping you find freedom.

I could not be more proud of Teresa. It seems whatever direction or insights I have ever offered her, she has taken to heart, put into practice, and was soon running circles around me! I hope you will enjoy her work as much as I do. I hope you will feel how much she cares about where you are and knows what keeps you from where you want to be.

Your journey starts now. Hope lives. I'm excited for what lies in store for you!

WENDY K. WALTERS
Author, Speaker, Mentor, Friend
wendykwalters.com

Your destiny is wrapped in becoming a vessel through which the love of God can flow unbruised and unfettered— completely free from strongholds that hinder you.

WENDY K. WALTERS

AUTHOR'S NOTE

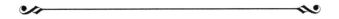

As Christians, we seem to have one huge disconnect. There are core truths about God we say we believe, but really don't because our actions don't reflect the words we are speaking. This is a problem we need to solve, but it's difficult for us to know where to begin. We're too close to the issue.

Jesus was pretty clear when He said, "All who love Me will do what I say. My Father will love them, and we will come and make out home with each of them. Anyone who doesn't love Me will not obey Me. And remember, My words are not My own. What I am telling you is from the Father who sent Me."[1]

What Jesus was saying is the thing Grandma said many times, "Actions speak louder than words." So, why do we say one thing and do the exact opposite? If our actions don't line up with our words, we have bought into lies which have grown into strongholds which keep us from some of God's greatest treasures—His truth.

The chapter titles in this book are truths God settled in my spirit once I invited Him to break the strongholds I had allowed the enemy to set up. In each chapter, I walk you through the lie I believed and how the stronghold grew. In the final analysis, it is His revealed truth which breaks the stronghold and sets us free. When we experience His truth in any area we will be set free in that area.

ACTION STEPS

Where the rubber meets the road is always in the application of truth to our lives. I write books praying they will help you find the freedom you need. With that in mind at the back of this book, you will find the Action Steps section. Each chapter has seven thought-provoking questions, writing prompts or exercises to help you apply the information in the chapter to your life. To get the very most out of this book, you will want to work through these steps.

God longs to uncover and break the strongholds you've allowed to take up residence in your heart and soul. We must invite Him to do that. He won't force Himself on us, but He will put us in situations that make it apparent what we must do to move forward. Removing strongholds will help you take steps towards overcoming life-controlling habits that have you bound. Mine was sugar addiction. Yours may be different.

OVERCOMING

As others have read this book and given me feedback, I realize how I dealt with sugar addiction also applies to those who have any life-controlling or life-devastating issues. Whether it is pornography, control issues, infidelity, gambling, over-spending, work addiction, guilt, shame, cigarette smoking, alcohol, drugs, relationship issues, marriage issues, people-pleasing, rage or anything else you want to overcome but can't, this book will help you.

Writing a book always reveals many things to me about myself and with each book I get set free in new areas. What I've learned is, we never arrive on our journeys with God. We are constantly in the process of arriving. It's a journey to greater and more glorious things every day.

Jesus said it this way. "I have told you these things, so that in Me you may have peace. In this world you will have trouble. But take heart! I have overcome the world."[2] To overcome is definitely the goal.

CONNECTING

The Next Steps section tells you how to connect with me. Feel free to email me or connect on any of my social media platforms.

My website is the best place to find all of my resources. Under the weight loss tab, you can find my coaching resources. My weekly podcast episodes are under the podcast tab. Under the books tab, you can find the other books in my Sweet Series. Most of all, be sure to check out the free tab where I have materials to help you. I can't wait to meet you!

P.S. Don't miss the link for my free gifts just for you. You will find that in the Next Steps section at the end of the book.

1. John 14:23-24 NLT
2. John 16:33 NIV

"The Lord your God is in your midst, a Warrior who saves. He will rejoice over you with joy; He will be quiet in His love, making no mention of your past sins. He will rejoice over you with shouts of joy."

ZEPHANIAH 3:17 AMP

CHAPTER 1

MY STRENGTH COMES FROM GOD

I was sitting at the kitchen table in our small two-bedroom apartment. My husband, Roy, had just left for work. The sun was streaming through the east-facing picture window.

My Bible was open to the book of Matthew. My journal was ready, and my pen was in my hand. Then, I glanced over at the three remaining cinnamon rolls from those I had baked that morning. Roy had eaten two before he left for work. I had eaten three others so far, but I really wanted the rest.

Before starting my time with God, I decided to fill my stomach again. God wouldn't mind. He'd want me to get this out of the way before talking with Him anyway. I grabbed the rolls and a diet cola to wash them down and started reading in Matthew 17.

I like to read until something catches my attention. I read about the transfiguration, but no special insights came. I continued reading how the disciples couldn't heal a demon-possessed boy. The father brought him to Jesus, and Jesus healed him. Then in a private conversation, the disciples turned to Jesus and asked why they couldn't drive out the demon.

It was when I read Jesus' answer to them that God's flashlight illuminated the passage and the words went straight to my heart. Jesus replied, "Because you have so little faith. Truly I tell you, if you have faith as small as a mustard seed, you can say to this mountain, 'Move from here to there,' and it will move. Nothing will be impossible for you."[1]

I HAVE A LITTLE FAITH

As thoughts coursed through my mind, I began writing. "God, I have a little bit of faith. I also have a mountain of flesh on my body. How can this mountain be moved?"

To put things in perspective, it was 1977 and I weighed over 200 for the first time in my life. I was headed towards 250 and I didn't like it. Still, I loved cinnamon rolls, cookies, cakes, mashed potatoes, french fries, pizza, rich casseroles, hot rolls, chips and so much more.

The passage I was reading was about Jesus. He is the one who said if I had faith, I could move a mountain. I wanted my mountain to move. He was the one who could tell me how to get it done.

He didn't answer my question in an audible voice but in the sense of knowing deep in my heart and soul. I know the answer was straight from Him because it is not an answer I expected, had ever heard anywhere before or had ever thought about.

I wrote what He said in my journal. "Stop eating sugar. Eat more meats, fruits and vegetables. Stop eating so much bread." This was my lifestyle change plan straight from Jesus.

I didn't have to stop and think about what I did next. I wrote my answer to Him, "Nice plan, Jesus. If I could do that, I could lose weight, but I can't do that."

I didn't ask Him if He could help me with this plan. I didn't tell Him I'd think about it. I didn't decide if He was telling me to do this, He must have a reason. I simply said, "I don't need Your advice, after all, Jesus."

I didn't want to give up sugar. I didn't think I should have to give up sugar forever. I knew the Bible well enough to know as a Christian I am free to do whatever I want and if I want to eat sugar, then I'm going to eat sugar. Nowhere in the Bible does it say, "Thou shalt not eat sugar."

THE SUGAR CONUNDRUM

The conundrum I found myself in, though, was I wanted to lose weight and I knew eating too many foods containing processed sugar was one of my biggest problems. Still, I didn't want to give up those foods completely. More emphatically, I was sure I could not give them up. They were too intertwined with who I was.

For the next 30 years, I tried to lose weight by finding diets that curtailed sugar and most breads and focused on protein, meat, vegetables and fruits. On those diets, I could lose weight, but I never learned anything about how to change my lifestyle. I'd stay on the diet until I got to a goal. Then I'd celebrate by baking one of Grandma's delicious oatmeal cakes and eating as much of it as I wanted.

Doing this meant I would go off the diet and gain the weight back plus more. One bite of any concoction that contained processed flour and sugar would mean I would go back to the way I had always eaten.

JESUS, YOU'RE MEAN TO ME

The plan Jesus gave me felt like He was being mean to me. Why could I not eat sugar? Others could eat it and not gain an ounce. Life was not fair.

He made Himself clear and plain to me on that day. It's a day I will never forget. It's the day my loving Jesus gave me a lifestyle change plan designed especially for me, but I thumbed my nose at Him and walked away. Even by this time eating sugar had become more important to me than following Him. I had no clue I would become more than twice the size I was then before I finally implemented His plan.

I didn't know I was already living a lie.

I didn't know I was already living a lie. It was a lie that affected my entire life—body, soul and spirit. My soul is made up of my mind, emotions and will. Those contain my thoughts, feelings and desires which were all involved in helping me believe the lie I needed sugar to survive.

I was programming my body to want more sugar. If I'd been in my right mind and thought about it logically, I would see eating sugar was not good for me. I was gaining weight, taxing my body and setting myself up to develop diabetes, high blood pressure and many other diseases

I was denying the Holy Spirit access to all of me. I was choosing to allow a different spirit to control this one area of my life. I was blinded by a lie I had allowed to grow into a stronghold. I had certainly fed it often enough.

I didn't see overeating as a sin. I didn't understand damaging my physical body, which is the temple of the Holy Spirit,[2] was a sin. I also didn't understand even though I was saved, grew up in the church, attended church every Sunday morning, Sunday night and Wednesday night and followed all the church rules, I was still very capable of not only sinning but allowing a stronghold of sin to take over a part of my life.

I'd heard a lot of sermons about alcohol, drugs, dancing, premarital sex, even the dangers of secular music, but there was never one sermon about overeating. It was not on the list of my church's do-nots, which reminds me of the word donuts. Donuts was definitely on the church do list. They were what got me there early every Sunday morning.

> My reasons for wanting to lose weight were purely selfish.

When I asked Jesus how to move my mountain of weight, it wasn't because I was convicted it was a sin. It was because I saw my weight as an inconvenience. None of my clothes fit and I didn't have money to buy new ones. Plus, I didn't want to look like a fat blob. My reasons for wanting to lose weight were purely selfish as were my reasons for eating whatever I wanted whenever I wanted it.

I'm surprised Jesus even answered such a selfish prayer. He answered, though, because He had a vested interest in what I was doing to myself. He gave me the right answer, I just didn't realize the depth of the question I had asked. If I had known then what would eventually happen to me, all the difficulties, missed opportunities, pain and disease I had opened the door to, maybe I would have listened to Him. Sometimes, though, the best lessons are learned through experiencing our failures and brokenness.

I needed to understand what God was trying to tell me. I had asked Him many times to show me why I couldn't do what He wanted me to. Then one day I was reading the Bible and a verse I had never paid attention to jumped out at me. "Could it be any clearer that our former identity is now and forever deprived of its power? For we were co-crucified with Him to dismantle the stronghold of sin within us, so that we would not continue to live one momentlonger submitted to sin's power."[3]

It seemed so plain. I was shocked I'd never seen it before. **Before we come to Christ, Satan owns us.** Before we come to Christ, Satan owns us. We have to do what he says. We are in bondage to him. We have a stronghold of sin. When we become Christians, our old self dies, just like the picture baptism gives us. Our sins are buried in the water and we are raised to walk no longer having to listen to the devil. Jesus sets us free to choose. We are not under Satan's control. We can make different choices.

When we come to Christ, He wipes our slate clean of the sins we have committed. They are thrown into the deepest ocean.[4] They have been separated from us as far as the east is from the west.[5] God doesn't even remember what we've done.[6] Our past is in the past. We might remember, but as far as God is concerned, we're ready to start over. He declares us righteous because we have embraced and identified with His Son.

What has been removed from us is the obligation to sin, but the tendency or the urge to sin has not been removed. Sin's power is only removed when we walk with God and receive His dynamic power. It's broken when we choose to follow God. We do this by walking in His Spirit, being in constant communication with Him, listening to what He says and following Him in obedience. It doesn't happen automatically. We must choose Him by our actions.

> You cannot break a stronghold until you define it.

For any stronghold to be broken, I have to identify the stronghold. I can't break something undefinable. I went for years believing my desire to consume sweets and high carbohydrate-laden foods was normal. It wasn't a sin. It was just the way I was created. When I saw what I was doing was flagrant disobedience to God and still didn't give it up, I knew what was going on was bigger than just a little issue.

It was deeper than a lie: it was a stronghold. I had erected a prison inside me which I continued to build every time I dieted and tried to curtail eating sugar. I could lose weight, but I always gained it back plus more when I began eating sugar again. Then the evil one would whisper, "See, you can't give up sugar." I was caught in a prison of my own making.

The weapon against a lie is always the truth. When truth stares me right in the face, it's difficult to deny. I was in the super morbidly obese category. I had diabetes, high blood pressure, congestive heart failure, could barely walk and a cardiac surgeon had given me five years to live.

It was the beginning of finally facing the hard truth. What I was eating was killing me. I still wasn't ready to give up sugar, but I did go on another diet. The stronghold was not broken, though, until I understood I have the power to give up sugar. This power was given to me by Jesus Christ because He has all authority. For years I thought I didn't have a choice. I had to give into my thoughts, feelings and cravings. I was powerless over them.

In my humanity, I am powerless over sugar, but because I am joined to Jesus, I have a secret power I had not yet learned how to use. "Since you are now joined with Jesus, you must continually view yourselves as dead and unresponsive to sin's appeal while living daily for God's pleasure in union with Jesus, the Anointed One."[7]

My union with Christ is like a supernatural power generator just waiting for me to plug in. The way I plug into His power is not a secret. It's written in plain language in His Word. It is counter-intuitive especially to the modern-day culture which tells us we are strong, and we can overcome anything. We just have to put our willpower to it. God, though, doesn't work this way. He has a better plan.

WEAKNESS REVEALED

When I admit to God, I am weak in my human strength and surrender the area I am gripping tightly, I finally plug into His supernatural Holy Spirit power generator called grace. When I do this, I have more than enough strength, more than enough ability, more than enough anointing and more than enough power. Until then, the power is simply sitting there waiting for me to claim it.

"God has said to me, 'My grace is sufficient for you, My lovingkindness and My mercy are more than enough—always available—regardless of the situation; for My power is being perfected and is completed and shows itself most effectively in your weakness.' Therefore, I will all the more gladly boast in my weaknesses, so that the power of Christ may completely enfold me and may dwell in me.

"So I am well pleased with weaknesses, with insults, with distresses, with persecutions, and with difficulties, for the sake of Christ; for when I am weak in human strength, then I am strong, truly able, truly powerful, truly drawing from God's strength."[8]

I was able to choose to rest in the complete strength of Christ.

When I understood it was natural for me to be weak, it made all the difference in the world. When I accepted my weakness, I stopped trying to cover it up by running to every diet in the world. Then I was able to choose to rest in the complete strength of Christ. This is when I could finally do all things through Christ who gives me strength.[9] It's very simple and extremely difficult at the same time because we are taught to never admit our weaknesses.

I've learned my human strength only lasts so long. I could give up sugar for about nine months before I had to have another hit of my drug of choice. Surrendering my will to God and allowing Him to be my strength has made all the difference in the world.

It is only possible to break mental strongholds when we rely completely on the life-changing power of the Holy Spirit. I knew this long before I applied it to my situation. Right out of college, I was in a growing young adult group at my church. Bonnie, a co-leader of the group, taught us many melodies set to scriptures. The one I loved was Psalm 121 in King James Version.

When both of my children were born, this is the song I used as a lullaby. I wanted to make a lasting impression on them that God is their help and strength. If we truly surrender to His leading, He guides us in ways we could never imagine, guess or request in our wildest dream. He's not bossy or pushy about what He knows is the best for us. He just works in gentle ways with us, showing us the truth through His Holy Spirit working deeply within us.[10]

> Strength is not something we conjure up on our own own. It's a Person we submit to completely.

These words are for every person who longs for God to help them break free of the strongholds which have them bound. Power and truth are in these words. Our strength comes from God and Him alone. It's not something we conjure up on our own. It's a Person we submit to completely.

"I will lift up mine eyes unto the hills, from whence cometh my help. My help cometh from the Lord, who made heaven and earth. He will not suffer thy foot to be moved: He that keepeth thee will not slumber. Behold, He that keepeth Israel shall neither slumber nor sleep.

"The Lord is thy keeper: the Lord is thy shade upon thy right hand. The sun shall not smite thee by day, nor the moon by night. The Lord shall preserve thee from all evil: He shall preserve thy soul. The Lord shall preserve thy going out and thy coming in from this time forth, and even for evermore."[11]

God and God alone is my strength. When I follow Him I can do anything because He is giving me power. I gave up foods with processed sugar and gluten. It didn't happen overnight. It was a process that resulted in my total lifestyle change—body, soul and spirit.

The stronghold which says I'm not strong enough to give up sugar has been broken in Jesus' name. All praise and honor and glory go only to God. He is where my strength comes from.

ENDNOTES

1. Matthew 17:20 NIV
2. 1 Cor. 6:19 NIV
3. Romans 6:6 TPT
4. Micah 7:19 NIV
5. Psalm 103:12 NIV
6. Hebrews 8:12 NIV
7. Romans 6:11 TPT
8. 2 Corinthians 12:9-10 AMP
9. Philippians 4:13 NIV
10. Ephesians 3:20 MSG
11. Psalm 121 KJV

"I look up to the mountains; does my strength come from mountains? No, my strength comes from God, who made heaven, and earth, and mountains."

PSALM 121:1-2 MSG

CHAPTER 2

GOD IS MY GOD

Everything I had tried in order to lose weight and keep it off had failed. I had gotten to the point I didn't even care if I lived or died. It felt like I wasn't living when I was super morbidly obese. As a last-ditch effort to lose weight, I made a really bad decision which I don't recommend for anyone.

My doctor said the only hope for me to lose weight was to have weight loss surgery. It was touted as the cure for obesity. The minute I woke up from surgery I knew I had made a mistake, but the irreversible deed was done. The first year I was mad at myself and everyone connected with the surgery. The only thing it did for me was reveal how big of a sugar addict I really was.

I did lose weight, but only because the size of the stomach created during the surgery meant I couldn't eat much of anything for the first six months. Certain foods gave me esophageal spasms, which felt like food was stuck in the back of my throat. Sugary foods made me sick. I was mad I couldn't eat them. The surgery didn't fix me. It tortured me and made me one extremely angry woman.

I was so mad I found ways around the restrictions. I began drinking diet soda, which is something I wasn't supposed to do because it stretches out the small stomach. I didn't care. I thought I needed diet soda to live. I wanted my fix even if it only mimicked sugar.

To stop eating sugar for an entire year had worked for me to lose weight, but I still hadn't dealt with my sugar and food addiction.

About a year later I found I could begin eating small soft candies. Eating them one at a time all day long didn't make me sick.

I was once again putting weight back on quickly. With processed sugar in my system, I was back to feeling how I'd felt before which seemed normal to me. To stop eating sugar for an entire year had worked for me to lose weight, but I still hadn't dealt with my sugar and food addiction. They were even more entrenched because I knew what it felt like to not be able to eat sugar. I was more determined than ever to keep my supply always handy, even if I had to hide it.

WEIGHT LOSS SURGERY LIE REVEALED

There is a reason why some bariatric surgeons mandate that patients go through a food addiction recovery program before weight loss surgery. Rob Cywes, MD, Ph.D., bariatric surgeon and addiction management specialist, speaking at 2020 Quit

Sugar Summit[1] explained as many as 85 percent of weight loss surgery patients gain the weight back in two years if they have not gone through food addiction recovery before having surgery.

I saw this happening with those who had surgery around the same time I did. As I talk with my coaching clients who have had the surgery, I hear the same kind of stories. We are very inventive. We will find ways to continue to eat what we want when we want it and however much we want unless we accept and own our foundational lies. Until then, we will fight to preserve those lies.

I know well the push and pull conundrum Paul describes. "I want to do what is good, but I don't. I don't want to do what is wrong, but I do it anyway."[2] Even though I'd lost weight, I still wanted to eat sugar. I couldn't stop myself. Rationally and cognitively, I knew it wasn't good for me, but emotionally I wanted it anyway.

> Rationally and cognitvely, I knew it wasn't good for me, but emotionally I wanted it anyway.

I didn't realize it at the time, but this is a spiritual issue. I wanted to lose weight, eat healthly food and exercise but no matter what diet I went on, even if I lost weight, I couldn't seem to keep it off. I didn't want to go back to eating whatever I wanted to eat whenever I wanted it, but I always did.

What was so confusing to me is why I did this when I really, really, really wanted to lose weight. It was because I really, really, really wanted to eat what I wanted as well. It was so ingrained in me that even when I did the monster fix of weight loss surgery, I still found ways to eat what I wanted. My foundational lie was stubbornly in place.

Paul recognizes there is another power operating inside him fighting against what he knows is right. This other power is an unwelcome intruder in his humanity, his flesh, his body. This is an agonizing or miserable situation. If left to himself, he will align with things that lead to sin or disobedience to God.[3]

This was definitely what was happening with me because God had clearly told me what He wanted me to do years ago. Paul acknowledged because of Jesus' sacrifice on the cross God's mighty power provided a way out of the pull sin had on him. Jesus had renewed Paul's mind. Paul had to make sure his renewed mind was totally submitted to God.

LIVING BY THE SPIRIT

I had accepted Christ when I was seven. I couldn't understand why I couldn't access His mighty power to triumph over the sin which so easily seemed to entangle me.[4] I had Jesus, but my life didn't change significantly when I accepted Him at such a young age. I hadn't grabbed hold of the total breadth of what living for Him meant.

I didn't understand the Spirit of life flowing through the anointing of Jesus had already liberated me from sin and death. Clothed with humanity, Jesus gave His body to be the offering for my sin. Every righteous requirement of the law was fulfilled by Him living His life in me. I am free to live, not according to my flesh, but by the power of the Holy Spirit.[5]

Jesus overcame sin and death. Jesus will lead me to do the same, but I still have to make the right choice every day. I can follow Christ and live by the power of the Holy Spirit or I can choose to live according to my selfish, fleshly desires which results in sin and death.

All ten of the foster teens and young adults we have had in our home were living according to their flesh, even the ones who would listen to us and try to follow our simple rules still had their moments. This experience helped me understand this concept so much better.

Our flesh is the default pattern of our lives. "If left to myself, my flesh is aligned with the law of sin."[6] Satisfying our desires is what we will always go back to even if we have accepted Christ. It's like someone has given us a gift certificate, but we have never activated it. It won't be of any good to us unless we choose to buy something with it.

> We have to activate our desire to live for Him by committing to live according to the Holy Spirit's power.

When we accept Christ, we receive the Holy Spirit, the power which raised Christ from the dead.[7] We have to activate our desire to live for Him by committing to live according to the Holy Spirit's power. Until we commit to doing that we will still be back in the confusion and conundrum of Romans 7:19.

I was stuck there for many years, but I also desperately wanted to activate the full power of the Holy Spirit in my life. To do this, I was going to have to surrender everything to God even the foods I loved.

Russ Hardesty, a friend and counselor, was holding an informational meeting for a new group he was forming for individuals with harmful life patterns. There were many there with different problems like alcohol, drugs, pornography, overspending and food issues. I was gaining weight but wasn't admitting it. I was just going to support him. I didn't expect any personal change to come from the experience. I was living in denial and thinking I didn't need any kind of transformation.

Russ shared his story of being sober from alcohol for over 20 years. Alcohol has never been my problem. My paternal grandfather was an alcoholic. I promised Dad I would never drink alcohol or become addicted to anything. I kept the promise with alcohol. I was about to learn I hadn't kept the not being addicted part.

All of a sudden, I heard Russ say something which felt like it was meant just for me. The words seemed to come out of the blue and unattached to his story. He said, "Alcohol is one molecule away from sugar. Alcohol is liquid sugar." Those words grabbed me and wouldn't let go. He had my total attention.

I had heard enough to know if he had not gotten sober, he probably would have lost his job, his family and maybe even his life. He made a logical, rational decision to give up alcohol and then he had to learn how to walk out his journey one day at a time.

BONA FIDE, DIE-HARD SUGAR ADDICT

The truth hit me square in the face. I am like an alcoholic only with sugar. I crave it all the time. I can't stop eating foods that have processed sugar in them even after I have had a difficult, body-altering surgery. I can't stop eating them even though I know a cardiac surgeon has told me I will die if I don't keep the weight off. I am a bona fide, die-hard sugar addict.

At this time, I hadn't heard anything about sugar addiction. Social media wasn't a thing yet. The internet was just starting to invade our lives. I had never personally heard the words sugar addiction. However, right then I knew beyond a shadow of a doubt I was a sugar addict, even if it wasn't something any experts recognized as an issue. At the end of the meeting, I asked, "Can a person be addicted to sugar?" Russ looked me in the eyes and said, "You can be addicted to anything which controls you."

> Sugar controlled me. It mastered me. It called the shots in my life.

Those words sealed it for me. Sugar controlled me. It mastered me. It called the shots in my life. It told me what to eat, when to eat, how much to eat and never to stop eating. It made me feel better for a minute, then I needed more to get the same feeling. It controlled my spending habits, what I cooked and what I bought at the grocery store. It was one reason I still had credit card debts to pay off because I was always buying larger-sized clothes to accommodate my weight gain.

Finally, I saw what had happened. I had willingly allowed sugar to put me in bondage. It started as something fun to do like baking cookies with Grandma. It became a comfort to bake and eat cookies to dampen any thought or emotion I felt.

I saw how I began to buy into the lie which said eating my emotions away was better than trying to figure out how to deal with them. I saw how sugar had cozied up to me and made me feel better. It made me feel like I couldn't live without it, just like a manipulative lover might. All the time sugar was a tool of evil out to destroy me.[8]

At the same time, I saw how I had allowed my mindset of I cannot live without comfort foods to become a prison in my life. Setting myself free from its grip was not going to be easy. I was in a spiritual war. It was not going to be enough for me to go on another diet. I was in a battle for my very life.

I knew I couldn't fight this battle with weapons of the world. I had to have divine power to break and utterly destroy the stronghold which got me to this place. I had to change my mindset, stop arguing with God and stop thinking I knew better than He did. I had to take every thought captive in obedience to Christ.[9]

In a moment of clarity, I realized what I had been doing was rebelling against God. I was following what my flesh, my appetite, my stomach wanted rather than what God wanted. This realization brought me to my knees.

"For, as I have often told you before and now tell you again even with tears, many live as enemies of the cross of Christ. Their destiny is destruction, their god is their stomach, and their glory is in their shame. Their mind is set on earthly things."[10]

TIME FOR SURRENDER

I was driving home after the meeting by taking country roads. I needed time to think and pray. I pulled off to the side of the road and cried out. "God, I see now how the lie I have been living relates to You. I believed the lie that I have to have sugar to survive. I have set sugar, the foods I crave and my appetite up as my god instead of You.

"Right now, in this minute and this place, I surrender sugar to You. I don't know how I'm going to do this. I know I can't do it like I did before. I want to learn how to give it up for good. I no longer want sugar to be my god. I want to follow only You."

This was my come-to-Jesus moment. It was as real or even more real than my salvation experience. I was a grown woman facing the results of my sin and rebellion against God.

There had been many times in my life when I told God I'd give up sugar, but I never meant I would give it up for the rest of my life. This was the first time I accepted when God says, "Stop," He means, "Stop." He doesn't mean to stop eating sugar for a little while and then go back to it. He doesn't mean stop eating sugar except when my daughter gets married and a piece of wedding cake is calling my name. He doesn't mean to stop eating sugar all year long, except on my birthday. When He says, "Stop eating sugar," He means, "Stop."

> This was my come-to-Jesus moment. It was as real as my salvation experience.

I knew what God wanted for me was a total lifestyle change. This would mean more than changing how I ate. I had to work on how to manage my emotions, how to change my thought patterns and how to recognize the spiritual lies I believed which I had allowed to grow into strongholds. To break those strongholds, I had to allow God to open my eyes and my heart to His spiritual truths.

Buried in all of these lies was a basic truth about God I had been missing. God is God. He is a jealous God because He knows when I put anything as more important than Him it will eventually destroy me. He kept calling me back to Him. He never gave up on me even though I so easily sold out to the god of my appetite. I covenanted with things I thought helped me, instead they were killing me, no matter how slowly.

God knew my issue with sugar and comfort foods would put me in an early grave if I kept eating them. He knew my love affair with sugar would only end in heartache. Even though I was stubborn, He never gave up on me.

> God knew my love affair with sugar would only end in heartache.

God loves me with a relentless love. It was because of His love He kept showing me the dangers of the path I was on. He wasn't being mean to me when He told me to stop eating sugar. He was trying to save my life. Instead, I was lost in my own lie.

All along His truth was right there in plain view. He had told me the truth many times, but every time I turned my back on Him. By my disregard for His instruction, I said, "If You're going to tell me no then I am free to not listen to You."

He will not violate the right He gave me to make my own choices. Still, He always gives me clear instructions regarding what He wants. He gave me a multiple-choice question along with the answer, but I still had a hard time passing the test of obedience.

"Today I have given you the choice between life and death, between blessings and curses. Now I call on heaven and earth to witness the choice you make. Oh, that you would choose life, so that you and your descendants might live! You can make this choice by loving the Lord your God, obeying Him, and committing yourself firmly to Him. This is the key to your life."[11]

Not only did He give me the right choice, He told me how to make the choice. It's by obeying Him and committing myself firmly to Him. When I do what I know He's asking me to do, then and only then, have I correctly chosen life. My actions reveal my true choice.

This is the antidote to the lie I was believing. When confronted with this scripture I would say, "I choose life." In reality, I was choosing death by eating what I wanted whenever I wanted it. I had chosen to tell myself I needed sugar and comfort foods to survive in the world as a Christian. I had kicked God off the throne of my life and set all the comfort foods I loved there instead.

If I truly choose life, then I am choosing to be obedient to God.

The truth God began to unfurl in front of me is He and He alone is God. He must be first in everything I do. If I truly choose life, then I am choosing to be obedient to Him.

Even though it felt like a magnificent secret He revealed just to me, it wasn't. It was a truth that has been there for centuries. I just had to make the determined choice by living my life in full accord with all He has for me.

One of the first steps was to be willing to say God is my God and then put Him first in my life. This was just the beginning. I had more strongholds to confront, more areas to heal and much more to learn about how to walk out my journey allowing God to be God of every part of my life.

ENDNOTES

1. https://www.quitsugarsummit.com
2. Romans 7:19 NLT
3. Romans 7:22-25 NLT
4. Hebrews 12:1 NIV
5. Romans 8:1-4 TPT
6. Romans 7:25 TPT
7. Romans 8:11 NLT
8. John 10:10 NIV
9. 2 Cor. 10:5 NIV
10. Philippians 3:18-19 NIV
11. Deuteronomy 30:19-20 NLT

WITH GOD ALL THINGS ARE POSSIBLE

"We don't have money to keep buying you new clothes every time we turn around," Mom said to me when I was in grade school. "You're growing too fast."

When she'd say things like that, I'd feel like I'd done something wrong. I felt guilty every time I grew an inch and needed different clothes, shoes or a coat. There was no one to hand clothes down to me. Mom tried sewing a few things, but she just wasn't any good at it. This meant she had to find money in our tight family budget to buy things for me.

When she complained about me needing bigger clothes, I thought I needed to stop growing, but I was a kid. At nine years old if I wasn't growing it would indicate something was wrong.

I wasn't fat, but I was always taller and a bit bigger than the small, petite, pretty, popular girls in my classes at school. I had already started puberty and needed different underwear in addition to larger-sized clothes. I hated it because all the changes happening in me meant I was a huge inconvenience to my family.

GAINING WEIGHT

One day I overheard Mom and Grandma talking about the clothes I had in my tiny closet. It was the middle of the school year. We didn't buy clothes except at the beginning of school, but I couldn't wear any of the dresses in my closet and the shoes were hurting my toes. She and Grandma were having me try on clothes to see if they fit.

I was in the bathroom and heard Mom say to Grandma, "She just keeps gaining weight. She's in husky sizes. I can't find anything in girls' sizes to fit her and women's sizes don't work yet. If they fit in the waist, they are way too big in the top. She's got to stop gaining weight, but it's like she just can't stop eating."

> I can't lose weight. I will never be able to lose weight.

Mom's voice was a frustrated whisper. Grandma said, "It's nothing to fret about. Kids have to eat. God gave her a healthy appetite. She can't help gaining weight. She needs to grow."

Out of that conversation, I assumed Grandma agreed with Mom that I can't stop gaining weight. I allowed what I ascertained as truth to begin to take root in me. What else could I do when the two maternal figures in my life agreed? It felt entirely like a truth. I can't lose weight. I will never be able to lose weight. It's impossible for me to lose weight.

It was true that as a child I couldn't lose weight. I was not meant to lose weight. I was designed to grow. I did not have the ability to figure out if what my Mom said was true. I certainly never thought it was a lie. When I perceived what Grandma said supported this, it became a solid truth.

The Bible says, "When I was a child, I talked like a child, I thought like a child, I reasoned like a child; when I became a man (or woman), I did away with childish things."[1]

I did not have the capacity to think or reason through what was true and what wasn't.

I did not have the capacity to think or reason through what was true and what was false. In most cases, children can go to their parents to learn the truth. Because Mom was emotionally ill, I didn't think I could ask her what she meant. I didn't want to ask Grandma or Dad because if they agreed with her, I was doomed.

I believed Mom. I had evidence to support what she was saying. I was growing, gaining weight and needing larger size clothes. I wasn't fat, but I was at least a size larger than most girls in my class. It became a belief of mine that it was impossible for me to lose weight.

In high school, I was in the marching band for one semester. An hour of early morning band practices every weekday for two months at the beginning of my sophomore year netted a 20-pound weight loss. It should have shown me I could lose weight if I exercised. Instead, I was just frustrated with having to get to school at seven in the morning because Mom wanted me to play in the marching band. I would have rather taken an art class.

After marching band, I put the weight right back on, especially with Thanksgiving, Christmas and New Year's Eve falling in line. Food, food, food and more food marked each special event. It was who we were. It was how I grew up. It further reinforced the idea that I can't lose weight. It's impossible.

IDENTIFYING LIES

When I became an adult, I still believed this lie because I saw it happen time and time again. I'd go on a diet and lose 100 pounds only to gain it back when I'd hit the goal because I'd start eating my comfort foods again.

I'd tell myself, "It's true. I can't lose weight. It's possible for others, but not for me. I am destined to remain fat for the rest of my life. It is impossible for me to lose weight." I had allowed this lie to become a full-blown stronghold in my life. Breaking it was going to take some work.

For God to get my attention with His truth on this subject, He needed to show me how untrue the statement I can't lose weight was. He had to jolt me into the reality of my predicament.

In 1999, I was in the hospital for a possible mitral valve replacement. I vividly remember the cardiac surgeon walking into my room and telling me, "You don't need heart surgery. You need to lose weight. Your heart was never designed to pump blood through a body of your size. You need to lose 100 pounds and keep it off or you will be dead in five years."

So, I lost 100 pounds by going on a high protein diet I'd been on before. Like all the other times, though, I began gaining the weight back after losing it. I kept it off longer, but I began eating sugar-laden foods again. The truth is, it's impossible for me to lose weight if I eat foods that contain processed sugar. When I start eating those kinds of foods again, I can't stop. They are very addictive to me.

DYING SWEETLY

Understanding the deeper reality behind this was right in front of me, but I did not know how to face it or fully embrace it. For many years I wallowed in this place of losing weight is impossible. Rooted in my childhood, this belief went deep and stayed until God brought me face-to-face with my problem.

This was when God revealed to me that I am a sugar addict. The truth hit me. The only way to get free from an addiction is to stop indulging in it. Every time I'd go on a diet where I gave up sugar and bread, I could lose weight. I just never saw it as something I'd have to do for the rest of my life. Understanding that felt like a tremendous weight was lifted from me, but in its place was the conviction of the Holy Spirit.

I didn't know how, but I knew I was going to have to get some help to understand how to give up sugar and bread. Although I felt the weight of this responsibility, I also understood if God had moved heaven and earth to show me this, He would also reveal to me how to make this monumental change.

> I knew I was going to have to get some help to understand how to give up sugar and bread.

God knew my tendencies. He knew my biggest weakness. He revealed it to me early, so I would not have to suffer through years of super morbid obesity. He was not trying to be mean to me by telling me not to eat sugar. He was trying to keep me from the one thing which would kill me quicker than anything else. I just didn't want to listen to the cure for my problem.

This stronghold had become a negative prophecy which the evil one repeated to me often. He even mimicked Mom's voice when he said it. "You can't lose weight. You're destined to always be fat. It's impossible so just stop trying."

When I felt like I had no way to stop the inevitable weight gain, I fed the feeling of hopelessness with the only thing I knew would quiet it and allow me to go about in a somewhat normal state of emotions. Comfort foods anesthetized my pain for a short time, then I needed more to get the same feeling.

When I came to the end of myself and totally surrendered to what God had been telling me, my life began to transform. The switch in my brain happened in an instant the moment I recognized the truth. The truth is I can lose weight if I stop eating sugar.

PHYSICAL OR SPIRITUAL WAR?

There were many times I stopped trying to lose weight because I could recount all the times it hadn't worked. The lie of I can't lose weight had become a well-entrenched stronghold to the point that seeing anything different about myself also felt impossible.

I know I'm not the only one who feels this way. I have women who come into my coaching group and then leave a week into the process because they once again believe they can't lose weight and feel like failures. They have been brainwashed to think only following a diet perfectly will help them. As a coach, I don't provide a diet. I help people learn how to change their lifestyles for true transformation. This involves every part of us—body, soul and spirit.

According to the online dictionary, the word diet means the kinds of food a person, animal, or community habitually eats. The second meaning is a special course of food to which we restrict ourselves in order to lose weight. We all are eating on some kind of diet. It might be the kind where we don't stop and think about what we eat, we just eat **We are all eating habitually in some fashion.** whatever our stomach or taste buds tell us to eat. Still, we are all eating habitually in some fashion. To lose weight, we have to change our habits.

All the diets I went on which worked to some degree were ones where I'd eat 1,000 calories a day (which I don't recommend for anyone) and greatly limit the types of foods I ate. I lost weight, but I never intended to do it forever. Habit change was not part of any diet I was on. Therefore, I would go back to how I had been habitually eating all my life. This is why I could never lose weight. I needed to change my habits. It felt impossible because I was in a war, but it wasn't a physical war. It was a spiritual war.

THE BATTLE

The fleshly, human desires we have collide with what God's Spirit wants for us and create a war in our minds. My physical desire to eat the foods which were making me gain weight was fighting against what God's Spirit wanted for me which was to be healthy in every area. The evil one was siding with my body to cause me to defeat myself.

Everything about me was hunkered down fighting along with Satan against God to preserve my right to slowly kill myself. My mind was a captive to the stronghold of I can't lose weight. My appetites and desires were fighting to keep eating all the things I thought made me feel better. My side of the war was being financed by the not so silent partner called the devil.

It was a very spiritual war, but it was one I had invited the evil one to join me in. I had done this from the time I was a child and believed the lie I couldn't lose weight. I reinforced it every time I tried and failed to lose weight.

My appetites and desires were fighting to keep eating all the things I thought made me feel better.

Our minds are complex and can think many things at the same time. They can want us to follow what we know God wants, but when we have allowed a stronghold to be formed in us and is connected to our appetites and desires, the evil one is sure he's won the battle.

To break this stronghold, I had to surrender to the power of the Holy Spirit to guide me. Step three of the 12 Steps of Alcoholics Anonymous says, "I made a conscious decision to turn my will and my life over to the care of God as I know Him." As a sugar addict, this means I need the guidance of God every single minute of every day.

If I am not in touch with Him, my life will be guided by my fleshly desires, selfish thoughts and unrealistic feelings. Surrendering to allowing Him to guide my life is much different even from the heart-felt emotional time I first surrendered sugar to God.

I had to commit to live my life in the ways of the Spirit guided by His power. I stopped living out of my thoughts, feelings and desires and started living by the power of the Holy Spirit. This is the place where strongholds begin to crumble. They cannot stand unless I stand with them. When I stand against them backed by the power of the Holy Spirit they are not just broken, they are shattered.

> We don't have to give in to what we think we want.

This takes consistent time with God, communicating with Him for every step we take. It means time in silence with Him where we just sit at His feet and listen for His voice. Most of the time we are too busy telling Him what we want to listen to what He's saying to us.

His Spirit of resurrection lives in us. He breathes life into us. This means our fleshly desires do not have to rule us. We don't have to live in obedience to what our fleshly desires tell us to do. We don't have to give in to what we think we want.

When we taste everything God offers which includes abundant life, we won't want to go back to something that is a very poor imitation of anything heavenly. **As** mature children of God we must be moved by the impulses of the Holy Spirit.[2]

TRANSFORMED LIVES

It's so simple, but we make it so difficult. God gave us free will. When we accept Him, we are finally free to follow Him. We have power over our flesh. Before we couldn't say no to things we had allowed to control us. However, if we have accepted Christ, we are no longer obligated to do the wrong thing. Daily living in the Spirit breaks the stronghold the evil one has over us.

"If you are living by the power of the Holy Spirit you are habitually putting to death the sinful deeds of the body, you will really live forever."[3] The operative word in the last sentence is habitually. It's not a one-time surrender. It is a daily surrender to Him. Spirit-led living leads us to transformed lives, but only when we are habitually choosing the right thing and habitually following how the Holy Spirit is leading us.

> We have access to the supernatural strength of God to overcome any obstacle.

Living Spirit-led is far from simple. We have accepted Christ, but this doesn't mean we won't be tempted. We will have to endure more temptation. At the same time, we know beyond a shadow of a doubt that we have access to the supernatural strength and power of God to overcome any obstacle.

"Never doubt God's mighty power to work in you and accomplish all this. He will achieve infinitely more than your greatest request, your most unbelievable dream, and exceed your wildest imagination! He will outdo them all, for His miraculous power constantly energizes you."[4]

All I had to do was follow Jesus, stay in communication with the Holy Spirit and trust God for the outcome. I began to not only believe but embrace and live out this truth. God's truth is the sledgehammer which will break strongholds to the point they are utterly destroyed. Lies are powerless in the light of God's truth. The truth trumps every lie.

GOD IS POWERFUL

I believed a lie that said I can't lose weight. Never in my wildest imagination did I ever think God could help me lose the weight I needed to lose. I thought even God wasn't big enough to help me. I thought I was beyond help.

God did just what Jesus said He could. "What is impossible with man is possible with God."[5] I tried losing weight on my own, but I couldn't. I tried going on diet after diet to lose weight, but I would only gain it back plus more. I believed a lie which said I couldn't lose weight. I thought it was just a part of me like brown eyes and freckles. I couldn't get rid of it.

God showed me how wrong I was to allow this lie to become a stronghold which kept me bound for too many years. He definitely did the impossible in my life when He helped me break this stronghold. It was just one of the ones propping up my addiction to sugar.

He is the God of the impossible and no one can tell me anything different. With Him all things are possible, even me losing an extreme amount of weight and keeping it off.

ENDNOTES

1. 1 Corinthians 13:11 AMP
2. Romans 8:14 TPT
3. Romans 8:13b AMP
4. Ephesians 3:20 MSG
5. Luke 18:27 NIV

"What is impossible with man is possible with God."

LUKE 18:27 NIV

CHAPTER 4

GOD DOESN'T CONDEMN FAILURES

It happened so fast I didn't know how to react. My 10-year-old daughter was in an all-day physical education event at our local university's field house, which happened to be in the middle of the campus not near any parking lot.

Like a good mom, I didn't just want to drop her off on a large college campus. I wanted to get her inside, signed up and then arrange to pick her up at the right time and place. This necessitated finding a parking place and trudging a mile or so with her to the correct building.

OK, no big deal. I needed exercise, but at my size, this was no easy feat. I was driven by love for my daughter and nothing else. We got there and got her to the right place. However, what happened on my very slow and laborious walk back to the car is forever etched in my memory.

I was focused on walking, not falling and just breathing when I heard a sound like mooing.

"Well, that's strange," I thought. "There are no cows around here."

When I heard it again, I looked back behind me to see three college boys on the other side of the street pointing at me, laughing and yes, mooing, again.

I gave them my best stare, turned and kept walking. They kept laughing and mooing. I felt like a failure. I was so glad my daughter was not with me. I didn't want her to feel like a failure because she had a mother who was a failure.

LYING THOUGHTS

Lying thoughts from the enemy immediately attacked me. "You deserve that. You are a failure. Look at you. You are a failure as a mom. You are a failure as a wife. You are a failure as a woman. You are nothing but a fat cow. Every single person who sees you wants to do the same thing those boys just did. They were just being honest with you."

In the midst of all of this I never once felt or thought what might have helped me which was, "Well, yeah, but Jesus loves me. He calls me His child. He accepts me. He calls me beautiful."

> Lying thoughts from the enemy immediately attacked me.

Instead, I felt God was secretly applauding those boys. Maybe God was even instrumental in their derision of me. This wasn't a new lie. I had already been telling myself this for years. One doesn't gain an enormous amount of pounds without feeling the weight of shame and the extreme sense of failure it brings.

Shame didn't start that day. It started as early as third grade when I was eight years old. It was the year my baby sister was born and the year I got glasses. Those two things happened close to the same time.

Every Friday morning, we had a time where we could share anything new which had happened during the week. Nothing new ever happened to me, so I was excited when I finally had something to share. Most of the kids would share things like getting a new toy, new clothes, a new bike or even a new house.

I was sure my news would be better than anything they had ever shared. Their new things all had to do with prestige. Mine was different. For the first time, I could read the blackboard. This was a big deal to me. The best thing, though, was my baby sister. Who could top that?

One of the popular boys shared how his dad had gotten a major promotion and they were moving to a new house. Then one of the other girls told how she had started dance lessons. I was still convinced my news would floor everyone.

FOUR-EYED FATSO

When my turn came, I nearly ran to the front of the class and said, "For the first time I can see the blackboard from my seat at the back of the class when I put on my new glasses." Then, I put on my red glasses with thick lenses. Today, we'd call them cat's eyeglasses because of the shape of the lenses.

Most every kid burst out laughing. They were pointing at me and one boy on the front row said, "Look at the four-eyed fatso." I slinked back to my seat fighting back the tears without telling the best news of all. They didn't deserve to hear it.

Mrs. Young[1] quieted the class and warned them of her rules which included not making fun of fellow students. Then, she quickly transitioned to teaching math. This was one of the first times I remember being ridiculed for being larger than the other kids.

My size made me self-conscious. I always felt I was fat because I was a little taller and bigger than the other kids. I didn't have fancy clothes like the popular kids, and I was no longer one of the smartest kids in the class.

Each grade had three classrooms—a low, middle and high class. Students were placed in the class depending on what grades they made the year before. I had made all E's in second grade, so I was in the high class. This meant I was in the class with many of the popular kids.

Being in the smart class meant I was graded according to others in the class. Most of the other kids expected to make all E's. In this class, I would be lucky to make M's which was average. I hated being me. I hated being fat. I hated not having nice clothes. I hated not being as smart as everyone else. It all made me feel like a failure.

GROWING UP BELIEVING A LIE

Standing in front of my third-grade classroom and being ridiculed was just the beginning of a lie I believed for most of my life. As I was growing up there were many times this stronghold of feeling like a failure and hating myself for some reason or another got triggered.

When we don't like ourselves, we don't think we are worth investing the time and energy to make changes. We don't believe there could be anything worthwhile inside us. When we hate ourselves, we don't even feel like we have the right to live. When we feel like failures, it makes us want to crawl in a hole and never come out.

We are sure whatever great gifts, talents and skills God put inside us when He saw us before we were being formed in utter seclusion,[2] must have been given to someone else. We begin to believe we've used up our gifts by eating ourselves into oblivion. This grows into there is no hope for us. We would be better off dead, even our family would be better off if we weren't here. We're failures.

The one thing we think we are doing for ourselves is the thing which is causing our demise.

This becomes a very scary stronghold. It doesn't seem like a lie because we think it's true. It has taken us over and until we recognize it as a lie, it will be nearly impossible for us to go forward. We have to learn how to love ourselves but when we are caught in this lie, we don't believe we are worth loving because we are big fat failures.

To feel like we aren't failures, we have to make ourselves indispensable to someone. As a result, we try to take care of everyone else. We put everyone else's needs, wants and desires ahead of our own. We put our needs last and let ourselves go. The one thing we think we are doing for ourselves is the thing which is causing our demise. Our one desire, our one pleasure in life is eating whatever we want whenever we want it.

We are rewarding ourselves for trying to help everyone else and getting nothing but more people wanting a piece of us.

We ruin our health because we are still trying to get people to approve of us. At the root of the hatred of ourselves is the desire for people to like us. We will do almost anything to make this happen.

I was not a failure and I was not fat, but both felt like truths when I heard the entire class laughing. I won't say the rude third grader was the devil, but the devil sure used him to set up a foundational lie in me. "You're a four-eyed fatso" played on repeat in my mind for years after.

TRIGGERED THOUGHTS

It's interesting how some incidents trigger thoughts like, "I am fat. I am nothing." These thoughts then go through our conscious minds and are archived in our subconscious. My brain is the physical part of me where my conscious thoughts are stored. There is also another section of my brain called the subconscious where everything I've ever felt, thought, desired or done is stored.

My brain is like my computer. The hard drive in my computer is like my conscious thoughts. They can be readily accessed for everyday functions. My subconscious is like a larger external hard drive. It is only accessed when I do a specific search there to find something. These subconscious thoughts can lie dormant for years waiting for some incident to trigger them to come to our minds.

I can be an intelligent, well-educated adult knowing exactly what I should eat, how I should move and the proper amount of sleep I should get. I can be losing weight and doing everything right. Then I'm walking down the street and some freshman boys make a derogatory noise and I'm back in the third-grade classroom with a rude boy calling me a four-eyed fatso.

This can be the very moment I go off my eating plan. I don't connect the dots because as quickly as the memory is retrieved it goes back into my subconscious waiting for another time when the enemy calls it up to make sure I am still believing the lie which shouts, "You are a failure."

> Feelings speak louder than cognitive thoughts.

I am afraid to dig deep to try to get the root of my problem. Instead, I prefer to overeat, so I don't have to think about being a total failure. I try to quiet my thoughts, memories and emotions by stuffing them with food. Instead of facing my problem and getting to the root of my issue, I choose to act on my selfish desires to eat whatever I want whenever I want.

LIES AND TRUTH

It's really difficult to understand how mindless words coming out of a child's mouth can set off a ripple effect that can snowball into me gaining an enormous amount of weight years later. It wasn't his fault, though. It was my perception, my negative self-image, which by age eight was headed downhill fast.

Feelings speak louder than cognitive thoughts. My thoughts are shifted by my emotions. My feelings used a third grader's words as a launching pad to build a stronghold of failure, shame and condemnation in my life. I was guilty of eating more than I should have. Even as a kid I'd sneak candy and cookies whenever I could.

Instead of asking God for forgiveness, repenting of my sin and turning around, I chose to wallow in shame and condemnation. I chose to believe the enemy's voice which said, "You are what you did. You are fat. You are shameful. You are a horrible donut monster. You are a failure. You should be ashamed of yourself, very ashamed."

Guilt says, "I have done something wrong," but shame says, "I am wrong." Shame is guilt turned inward. We are all guilty. There is not one person who has ever been born, except Jesus, who has never sinned. Sin is a fact of this life. It is easy to reconcile our guilt by simply asking for forgiveness. If we are truly repentant and confess our sins, then Jesus is "faithful and just and will forgive us our sins and purify us from all unrighteousness."[3]

> Failure, shame and condemnation become strongholds when we can't forgive ourselves.

If we don't confess what we've done or if we are not repentant, the evil one will help us internalize our guilt, which we turn into shame. It starts with him whispering to us we are what we have done. We feel guilty because we have not confessed and repented of what we see as something necessary to maintain our sanity.

Failure, shame and condemnation become strongholds when we can't forgive ourselves. The enemy keeps pounding it into our heads and reminding us that who we are will always be defined by what we've done. If we nurse and feed our negative thoughts about ourselves, they grow into full-blown strongholds. It becomes natural for us to fail because we believe we are failures. It's deeply embedded in us.

Shame followed me. I could never seem to shake it on my own. It was much later I learned grace is the trump card which does away with shame. Jesus is the only one who can play the right card for me.

The first thing many of us do when we feel we have failed is to invite condemnation and shame to flood over us. When the poor, poor pitiful me syndrome happens, instead of using it to propel us to do something about our plight, we bury our sorrows in ice cream, cake or whatever addiction pops into our minds.

This serves to make us believe we are failures once again. All along we haven't caught on to what the enemy is doing. He whispers nasty words of failure and shame in our ears because of our size. He tells us lies which sound so inviting. "I'm so sorry you are feeling sad, but I can help you. Just eat this cake and ice cream and you'll feel better in no time. Yes, you are a failure, but that's Ok. I've got the solution."

> Once the stronghold is firmly established, the addiction takes hold.

It becomes an endless cycle we don't see because we are so focused on what we desire, what we feel and what we think we want that we don't even bring God into the equation. We just assume this isn't a problem God would even care about.

We have become so comfortable with the voice of the enemy that we can no longer hear God's voice. We still love God, but in this one area, we have allowed the devil to talk us into erecting a stronghold of failure and condemnation. Once the stronghold is firmly established, the addiction takes hold. We feel we need it to survive because we cannot live in failure, shame and condemnation.

When we continue to return to unhealthy foods we know are killing us, the lies of the stronghold have become too heavy for us to carry. At this point, we become focused on what our physical bodies want instead of what we need. We have no desire to allow God to attack the stronghold by renewing our minds.

God, though, will never stop trying to get our attention. He knows for change to happen we must invite Him to do the work within us. It's the only way to be transformed and transformation is definitely what we want. "Fix your attention on God. You'll be changed from the inside out. Readily recognize what He wants from you, and quickly respond to it."[4]

We have to stop thinking like the world and start thinking like God.

The only way to be transformed is to allow the Holy Spirit to work on the inside of us. We have to stop thinking like the world and start thinking like God. This takes a total reformation of our thought processes. "Stop imitating the ideals and opinions of the culture around you, but be inwardly transformed by the Holy Spirit through a total reformation of how you think. This will empower you to discern God's will as you live a beautiful life, satisfying and perfect in His eyes."[5]

Transformation begins in the mind. This is good because when we become Christians, we have the mind of Christ which allows us to understand spiritual things we could never understand before.[6] This is a fundamental difference between us and those who don't have Christ.

God began to show me people in the scriptures who experienced failure and were transformed. They aren't difficult to find. Moses was a murderer. Abraham was a liar. Jacob was a trickster. Paul was a murderer. Rahab was a harlot. Gideon was a coward. The list could go on. Each of these learned from their mistakes and became better people.

David was another great man who was both a failure and a success. He had an affair with Bathsheba, got her pregnant and had her husband killed. Psalm 51 is a beautiful example of his truly repentant, transformed heart.

> Your abundant love is enough to wash away my guilt.

"God, give me mercy from Your fountain of forgiveness! I know Your abundant love is enough to wash away my guilt. Because Your compassion is so great, take away this shameful guilt of sin. Forgive the full extent of my rebellious ways and erase this deep stain on my conscience. I'm so ashamed. I feel such pain and anguish within me.

"I can't get away from the sting of my sin against You, Lord! Everything I did, I did right in front of You, for You saw it all. Against You, and You above all, have I sinned. Everything You say to me is infallibly true and Your judgment conquers me."[7]

We can feel David's anguish, pain and heartfelt repentance knowing what he did was not just a sin against others, but against God Himself. The key part of this, though, was he asked God to forgive him and do a complete restorative work within him.

"Create a new, clean heart within me. Fill me with pure thoughts and holy desires, ready to please You … Let my passion for life be restored, tasting joy in every breakthrough You bring to me. Hold me close to You with a willing spirit that obeys whatever You say. Then I can show to other guilty ones how loving and merciful You are. They will find their way back home to You, knowing that You will forgive them."[8]

We know David was a man after God's own heart even though he failed big time. He brought his failures to God and laid them on the altar. He asked for forgiveness and God forgave him. This is the only way David could go forward. He not only knew God would forgive him, he fully tasted of God's forgiveness. Shame was no longer an issue for him.

We don't refer to David as the adulterer and murderer. He is known best as King David, the giant killer, the man after God's own heart. David didn't see himself by the mistakes he made. He did not let shame keep Him from loving God.

> My failures remind me I don't want to fail again because my consequences can be grave.

Gaining the weight I did meant I was a huge failure. However, God never condemned me for my failures or called me a four-eyed fatso. He redeemed those failures. They have been some of my very best teachers. They have taught me I need to plan what I will do when tempted. When I do fail, I think through what I did and what I can do differently if in a similar situation. This way my failures aren't failures anymore because they have helped me learn how to have future successes.

My failures remind me I don't want to fail again because my consequences can be grave. Not because God would condemn me, but because my very body would. God knows this and so He leads me away from the things which will harm me.

There was a time even after I lost weight when all I could focus on was my failure. I kept telling God how sorry I was for my sin of rebellion against Him, for not listening to Him, for refusing to follow Him. I was grieving what I had done to God. Each time I could hear God saying to me, "Your sin is forgiven and gone. It is no more."

> I have been transformed and redefined by the power of the Holy Spirit.

I don't know the exact year when I quit mourning what I'd done, but I know it was when I changed my website, Facebook and Twitter headers to reflect the before picture of me as fading in the background.[9] It was intentional. It was my statement to the world which said, this person was me and in many ways is still a part of me, but she is not me now. She is a fading memory.

I have been transformed and redefined by the power of the Holy Spirit. It put the focus on who I am today, not what I did which represented a huge failure. This failure is a part of my past, but it is and always will be in my past.

Today I am a different person, but I remember the pain and anguish the old me went through. Even though it took me some time to accept, I know beyond a shadow of a doubt God has forgiven me for all my failures.

"We have been ransomed through His Son's blood, and we have forgiveness for our failures based on His overflowing grace, which He poured over us with wisdom and understanding."[10]

There are real spiritual forces at work in our desire for ice cream and cake. We can overcome those forces only by staying close to Jesus, listening to Him and following what we know He wants us to do.

God does not and never will condemn us if we are His. "Now the case is closed. There remains no accusing voice of condemnation against those who are joined in life-union with Jesus, the Anointed One."[11]

> Redeeming our failures is where God shines best in our lives.

This doesn't give us a license to continue doing whatever we want to do. However, His grace is there to rescue us every step of the way when we confess what we've done, repent and start over. He wants us to learn from our mistakes, leave them behind and go forward propelled by His grace power.

God doesn't shame us. We do that ourselves. Those college boys weren't the source of my shame. I was shaming myself with every bite I took of the foods I knew God had told me were not the best choices for me.

This is why we must understand the battle we fight is first spiritual. We are not perfect, but thankfully redeeming our failures is where God shines best in our lives. We are human and God is God. Only He knows what we need.

To get rid of the stronghold which says, "I am a failure." I had to crave peace more than I craved the foods I loved. I had to understand just because there are times I make a mistake, it does not mean I am a failure.

I had to renounce the lie that I am a failure. I declared I am more than a conqueror through Christ Jesus my Lord,[12] which is another of God's spiritual truths. No child of God can fail because God's grace covers us. All we have to do is ask for His forgiveness and learn from our mistakes.

Laughing at the ridiculousness of what we have allowed to almost kill us helps us not buy into the enemy's lies again. Two incidents made me feel like a failure. The lie I internalized then became a stronghold and I chose to use sugar to try to ease the shame and condemnation I felt. This almost cost me my life.

What started it? The childish taunt of being called a "four-eyed fatso" and some no-account freshmen boys acting like cows.

Could it get any more ridiculous than this?

ENDNOTES

1. Not her real name
2. Psalm 139:16 NLT
3. 1 John 1:9 NIV
4. Romans 12:2 MSG
5. Romans 12:2 TPT
6. 1 Corinthians 2:16 NLT
7. Psalm 51:1-4 TPT
8. Psalm 51:10, 12-13 TPT
9. See https://www.teresashieldsparker.com/; https://www.facebook.com/TeresaShieldsParker; https://twitter.com/treeparker
10. Ephesians 1:7-8 CEB
11. Romans 8:1 TPT
12. Romans 8:37 NIV

"So now the case is closed. There remains no accusing voice of condemnation against those who are joined in life-union with Jesus, the Anointed One."

ROMANS 8:1 TPT

CHAPTER 5

JESUS WANTS ME TO FOLLOW HIM

When I was five years old, I was convinced Mom was the most beautiful woman in the world. I remember sitting in the only bathroom in our house watching her put on makeup complete with red lipstick. I was mesmerized.

She had acne scars from when she was a child, so when she'd go somewhere, she put on foundation and then, powder. She seemed to transform into a princess right before my eyes. It amazed me. I loved watching it happen.

She didn't wear eye makeup, but she loved bright red lipstick. With her dark hair and trim body, she looked like a movie star to me.

"Mommy, can I wear some lipstick?" I asked.

She laughed. "You're too young for red, but maybe we'll get you some pink you can play with. Every little girl needs to feel beautiful." She smoothed my hair and then went back to finishing her makeup.

She had just applied her lipstick when Dad came down the hall to hurry us along. He was preaching at a small Pentecostal church in another town. It was his first time there.

He took one look at my beautiful mother and his face went white. "You need to take off the lipstick," he whispered urgently. "You can't wear red lipstick to church." The words were meant only for Mom, but I heard them too. I sat there with my mouth open watching Dad hurry off to find his good Sunday shoes.

VANISHING BEAUTY

Mom's face fell as she began to wash off the lipstick. She was sad and I was sad for her. Her beauty seemed to fade as the beautiful red color disappeared down the drain.

"Why does Daddy not like lipstick? It makes you look so beautiful," I asked.

"He thinks being too beautiful is sinful," was her emotionless reply.

"But why? Doesn't God like beautiful things?"

"Go get your shoes on and find your little white Bible. We don't have time to talk about it now."

In the car, I tried to continue the conversation with Dad. "When I get to be a big girl, I'm going to wear makeup," I said.

"No," he said matter-of-factly.

"Why not."

"Because it's not what good Christian girls do."

For some reason, that particular answer satisfied me at the time. After all, he was a preacher. He should know.

For the next 55 years, I didn't wear makeup. There were a few times as an adult I would go to makeup parties and buy makeup. However, I had never learned how to apply it correctly, so I felt inept. Mostly, I just used a little powder and lip gloss every once in a while.

After all, I was a good Christian girl.

As I got older, I began to understand Dad's issue with makeup, shorts, sleeveless shirts, low-cut dresses, tight-fitting clothes and even pants of any kind on women.

He felt it indicated a woman of loose morals who wanted to attract men. He had other rules which went along with those. He preferred I wear dresses all the time. When I was at home and playing outside, I could wear slacks or shorts if the weather called for it, but I was never to wear those kinds of clothes out in public.

Along with no makeup was no jewelry or anything to call attention to myself. He also preferred I wear my hair long and not cut it. He did not want me to go to movie theaters or dances. Also, what he termed as mixed bathing was off-limits. This meant no swimming with boys present.

The other rules included no cursing, no holding hands with boys, no smoking, no drinking and no drugs.

HIPPIE ERA

My high school years fell during the era of tie-died t-shirts, bell-bottom jeans, hippies, drugs, sex and rock and roll. Fortunately, it also was the rise of the Jesus Movement. As the daughter of a preacher, I didn't rebel to the extent I could have, but there was still part of me that wanted to slap a "Question Authority" bumper sticker on the back of my car.

Dad's rules were founded not necessarily in scripture, although he was a man of the Bible. They came from the headquarters of our denomination, which felt very out-of-touch with the times. I still wanted to wear makeup. I still wanted to wear jewelry. I still wanted to go to dances, even though I wouldn't have known the first thing about how to dance. Still, it sounded like fun.

Dad's version of being a good Christian girl boiled down to this: don't do anything which might entice a boy. Stay away from bad boys whose only desire is to have sex. Girls must do this by not wearing anything provocative or anything which would call attention to themselves.

Mom bought me a book to read about becoming a woman. She had one talk with me to ask if I had any questions. The book was confusing, but I wasn't going to ask her my questions. We just didn't have that kind of relationship. From the little she said I got the feeling if I became sexually active before marriage, it would be all my fault because I would have enticed some boy.

It's probably not what she said, but that's the way I interpreted it. With all the precautions and her indicating that this would be something terrible to happen outside of marriage, I wanted nothing to do with being "sexy."

PLAYING DOCTOR

I got the distinct message what boys might do to me would be all my fault. This was further enforced by an incident that happened when I was six years old. There was a boy in our neighborhood whom I'll call Adam.[1] He was a little older than me, but he and my brother, Randy, who was three, liked to play in the woods together.

One day Adam asked me if I'd like to come play in the fort he had built. It was in the woods next to his house which was several houses down from ours. He had never let me play in his fort before, so I was excited to be included. He said he wanted to play doctor.

I was thrilled because I had gotten a doctor's kit for Christmas. I ran inside and got it and then went with them to the fort. Adam told Randy to be the receptionist. I would be the patient. Adam would be the doctor.

"Here, Doctor," I said. "You can use my doctor's kit."

"OK, but I don't think I'll need it," he said.

GUARD AT THE DOOR

He told me to crawl inside the fort and for Randy to stay by the entrance unless other patients came. If they did, he was to tell Adam right away. I was naive and had no idea what was about to happen. He said first he had to examine me in detail. I thought this was where he'd use the stethoscope and tongue depressor.

No, this is where he began touching me, first by pulling up my shirt and pressing on various places saying, "Does this hurt here? Does this hurt here?" Each time I'd say no. I didn't feel like he was doing anything wrong until he pulled my shorts down and then my panties.

I realized what he was doing wasn't right, but I didn't know what to do or say to make him stop. God, though, was watching out for me because Randy came in right as Adam pulled my panties down and said, "Daddy is calling us to come home for supper." He took one look at what was happening and added, "Hurry up, Sissy. We don't want to be late."

I put myself together and ran home as fast as I could. During supper, Dad asked where we were because it had taken a while for us to answer. I said, "We were playing in the woods by Adam's house."

"Yeah, Adam built a cool fort in the bushes," Randy added.

"What were you playing?" Mom asked.

It seemed like an eternity of silence before Randy blurted out, "Adam pulled Sissy's pants down."

It felt like all the air was sucked out of our small five-room house. Dad looked at Mom. The look spoke volumes. I stared at my plate suddenly not hungry. Dad said, "We'll talk about this after supper."

THE PUNISHMENT

When supper was over, Mom told me to go to my room until they came to talk to me. It felt like I was in there for 100 years before they came in. It was Dad who spoke first. Mom was the disciplinarian in the family, and I was sure she would spank me later. What they did was far worse than any spanking.

"Your mother and I have talked and we have decided you are not to play at Adam's house or in any of the wooded areas. You may play in our yard if there are other kids out there playing ball or tag, but you are to stay away from Adam."

"Can Randy play with Adam at his house?" I asked. "Can he play in the woods with Adam?"

"Yes, he can, but it's off-limits to you."

Then he left and Mom tried to talk to me about places I should never allow boys to touch me. I wasn't listening to what she was saying. I was miffed because it felt like I got punished for something Adam did. Who would punish him? No one. Would Dad talk to Adam's dad? Probably not. Would he talk to Adam? I didn't think so. No, Adam got off free and I had to stay away from him, but who was going to tell him to stay away from me?

It seemed they thought this was all my fault. Was it? I didn't know, but I was determined not to be put in this kind of situation ever again.

As a teen, young adult and even for years after I got married, I did many things to make sure I didn't attract the wrong kind of man who might take advantage of me. In other words, I followed all the rules. I had to. It is what good Christian girls do. I have to follow the rules to be a good Christian. These included all the rules Dad wanted me to follow.

Overeating was never seen as being a bad Christian.

There was one rule Dad never had. He never had rules about how much we could eat. Overeating was never seen as going against God or being a bad Christian. As an adult, I did feel remorse for overeating, and I did feel like God wanted me to lose weight. I just couldn't wrap my head around how to do it and still eat the foods I loved.

Instead, I just worked harder and tried to do more good things for God. I knew what the scriptures said. I knew I was not saved by following rules or doing good works, but the concept of grace seemed so unnatural.

Grace, of course, is not natural. It's supernatural. God's grace is undefinable. The crazy thing is we think it can't be possible that God's not sitting up in heaven somewhere keeping score of all we've done right and wrong. God is not concerned about our scorecard. He's concerned about our hearts. If we've truly decided to live for Him, we will follow Him. It's all He wants from us.

"It was only through this wonderful grace that we believed in Him. Nothing we did could ever earn this salvation, for it was the gracious gift from God that brought us to Christ! So, no one will ever be able to boast, for salvation is never a reward for good works or human striving."[2]

Those words helped convince me God doesn't expect anything from me. I don't have to do anything to earn the salvation He freely gave me. Still, following all the rules was a stronghold in me for many years. I couldn't understand why the Creator of the universe would give the gift of His salvation to me without expecting something from me in return. There is only one answer. He gave me grace, undeserved favor.

> I couldn't understand why the Creator of the universe would give the gift of His salvation to me without expecting something from me in return.

He expects nothing in return, but He desires I love Him completely and follow Him without question. If I never do another thing for Him, He still loves me. I still have His grace poured over me. I am covered in His grace.

Because I love Him it is my heart's desire to never again be caught in mental strongholds which keep me from being free to follow Him. I know I don't have to earn my spot in heaven. I know following the rules is not what will help me spend eternity with Jesus.

When I began to see the rules I was taught to follow were not necessarily God's rules, it helped me uncover the truth. My parents were trying to keep me safe, but I took it as gospel truth this is how I should act, or God would think I wasn't a good Christian. I might not make it into heaven if I didn't follow the rules. So, I better do everything I can to make sure I'm doing enough to earn my way there.

TOUCHING HEAVEN

I remember several years ago watching a message by a well-known pastor. He had a measuring stick that went to the ceiling of the large auditorium. He likened this to the measure of how good a person was. He put himself at a certain point which indicated he was a good person.

He said, "If this is where I am, where is Billy Graham?" He put Billy a long way above himself. Then he asked the same question about Mother Teresa and he put her a bit above Billy.

The clincher came when he asked, "If this is where I am and maybe you too and this is where Billy is and Mother Teresa is here, where is Jesus?'"

Of course, Jesus was at the top of the chart. "And really He's far above even this," he said, "because Jesus is off the chart. No matter how many good works I've done or rules I've followed, I will never be where He is. He is beyond my reach. It would be like trying to touch heaven. I can't do it. I need Him to be the key to get me in."

All our righteous deeds are as filthy rags in His sight.[3] Because of this, God sent Jesus to be our righteousness. "We all have sinned and are in need of the glory of God. Yet through

His powerful declaration of acquittal, God freely gives away His righteousness. His gift of love and favor now cascades over us, all because Jesus, the Anointed One, has liberated us from the guilt, punishment, and power of sin!"[4]

We have no righteousness. Even our so-called good works are done with us in mind instead of God. We do them thinking they will make our heaven resume better, but no resume will ever get us in heaven.

The stronghold of feeling like I had to follow the rules to earn my place in heaven kept me spinning my wheels and not listening to what God wanted for me. I can never repay the debt Jesus paid for me. I can only love Him and out of love follow wherever He leads me.

I have no standing to get into Heaven except I stand on the righteousness and faithfulness of Jesus. "So now, because we stand on the faithfulness of Jesus, God declares us righteous in His eyes!"[5]

BREAKING THE RULES

In 2013 when I was finishing *Sweet Grace*, Wendy Walters, my writing mentor, advised me, "Get your hair done, learn to put on makeup, get your nails done and buy some new clothes. You need to feel beautiful so your inner beauty can shine."

I was 60 years old and had lost 250 pounds, but what she was asking me to do broke all Dad's rules. I felt like a duck out of water, but I realized it was time to break free of the constraints I had placed around myself. It was time I learned how to look like a woman.

My niece gave me makeup lessons. I found an awesome hairdresser and a great nail salon. I got some new clothes. I allowed myself to feel pretty for the first time. Finally, I was tapping into how God made me. I'm a strong, beautiful woman. I am not afraid. God's got my back.

Beyond my desire to follow Dad's rules, the fear I felt in stepping out and making myself more presentable is a fear thousands, maybe millions, of women feel. Many have more of a reason to have this fear than I did. It's a fear of what others might do to them, but it is also a fear of their own sexuality, a beauty so strong it naturally draws men to them.

This fear can become another stronghold, but we need not be afraid of who we are. If we are sold out to God and allow His Holy Spirit to lead us each step of the way, He will remind us when we cross the line. He made us sexual beings. It is a gift He gave us. Used appropriately in marriage, sexuality, combined with emotional and spiritual connection, becomes an intimate bond between husband and wife. Why are we so afraid of this beautiful gift?

Why are we so afraid of this beautiful gift?

We are afraid of the misuse of the gift, a burning desire we cannot quench. Fleshly desires come in all shapes and sizes. Jesus said, "Here on earth you will have many trials and sorrows. But take heart, because I have overcome the world."[6]

If Jesus could overcome this temptation, so can we. He gave up His divinity for the time He lived on earth as a human with flesh, blood and desires. He was tempted in all ways like we were but did not sin.[7]

Many times, we see Jesus pulling aside to commune with His heavenly Father. He had to get instructions. He knew as a human, His connection to the Father was what kept Him alive and gave Him the power to overcome the pull of the world.

We have access to this same kind of connection through the Holy Spirit. Jesus told His disciples the Holy Spirit is the one who will lead, guide, teach and comfort them.[8] The Holy Spirit lives in us and is the same power that raised Christ from the dead.[9] He can help us resist temptation if we will submit our desires and cravings to Him. These only control us if we give them control. If we ask Him, He will lead and guide us.

Walking with Him becomes a marvelous adventure in abundance.

Walking with Him, then, becomes a marvelous adventure in abundance.[10] By His very nature, God's Spirit is a never-ending source of strength, power, love, peace and abundance. He is everything we need right now.

I am thankful God revealed His truth to me. I don't have to follow rules. Jesus invites me to follow Him.

The stronghold which says I have to follow all the rules to be a good Christian is broken. I can go to a movie. I can wear jeans. I can wear jewelry. I can even wear makeup.

As long as I am following Jesus, He approves of me. He calls me beautiful no matter what.

ENDNOTES

1. Not his real name.
2. Ephesians 2:8-9 TPT
3. Isaiah 64:6 NIV
4. Romans 3:23-24 TPT
5. Romans 3:26 TPT
6. John 16:33 NLT
7. Hebrews 4:15 NIV
8. John 14:16-17, 26; John 15:26; John 16:13-14 NIV
9. Romans 8:11 NIV
10. John 10:10 NKJV

"Here on earth you will have many trials and sorrrows. But take heart because I have overcome the world."

JOHN 16:33 NLT

CHAPTER 6

GOD IS MY PROTECTOR

Fear is a stronghold the devil loves to set up in us. All he has to do is move all the players in place to set up circumstances that cause us to feel we are all alone. This leads us to believe no one, not even God can protect us.

When this happens, we either go crazy or we try to protect ourselves. I couldn't go crazy because I had already determined I never wanted to be like Mom, who had issues with manic depression. This left me believing I had to protect myself.

When I first started realizing I had developed a stronghold of self-protection, I knew it stemmed from an incident when I was 11 and was molested by a family friend. I'll call him, Fred.[1] I was at the place I considered the safest place in the world—my grandparents' two-story farmhouse.

Fred and his wife, Minnie,[2] were visiting from out-of-state. Minnie was Grandma's best friend in the whole world. Even though they lived far away, they wrote every week. They told each other everything. The highlight of Grandma's week was hearing from Minnie.

Fred and Minnie didn't come every year because it was a long drive. When they did come our extended family got together as often as possible to hear Fred's stories. He liked to tell tall tales. Some were true, some were out and out lies, but everyone laughed at what he had to say. He was loud, boisterous and the life of the party.

From the minute he arrived, he was pulling silver dollars out of all of the girls' ears. This was in exchange for sitting on his lap and kissing him. When the silver dollars ran out, he'd pull quarters out of our ears. The boys got silver dollars and quarters, too, but I don't remember what they had to do for theirs.

He pulled silver dollars out of the girls' ears in exchange for sitting on his lap and kissing him.

I distinctly remember having to kiss Fred for my silver dollar. He smelled like cigarette smoke. His face was scratchy and needed to be shaved. His lips were big and engulfing. It was nothing like sweetly kissing Papaw on the cheek. From as far back as I can remember, I didn't like having to kiss Fred. I endured it because a silver dollar was a big deal.

Minnie and Fred had been coming back every two years or so, but this year I noticed Fred was acting differently towards me. He insisted I sit on his lap numerous times for kisses and silver dollars. He was also hugging me strangely. His hands were straying to parts of my body Mom told me I should never allow any boy to touch, except my eventual husband. I thought maybe I was just imagining it and went inside to help Grandma. I was staying there that night.

The next day was Sunday and everyone was coming back for lunch after church. Grandma's house had two stories. Upstairs was three bedrooms. Downstairs was the kitchen, dining room, living room, Grandma and Papaw's bedroom and the only bathroom in the house.

I usually slept on the couch or a pallet down beside Grandma. I was afraid of Boo, the ghost I thought lived upstairs. Even though I was the oldest grandchild and the one who had made up all the Boo stories, I was still scared to sleep upstairs by myself in case the stories came true. Since Fred and Minnie were sleeping upstairs, Grandma thought I shouldn't be afraid to sleep there.

THE ROOM AT THE TOP OF THE STAIRS

I chose to sleep in the room at the top of the stairs. It was right above Grandma and Papaw's bedroom downstairs. It was summer and the windows were all open so I could hear Papaw pray with Grandma before I fell asleep. All was right with the world. I had no inkling of what was in store the next morning.

I heard the door open. I opened my eyes and briefly saw Fred sneak into the room. I quickly shut my eyes again willing them to stay closed and trying to make him think I was asleep. I began praying silently for God to make him leave, but he was still there. I could hear his footsteps as he walked up to the bed.

I didn't know much about things boys do to girls and nothing about what older men might do to younger girls. I knew if he had good intentions, he would have thrown the door open and announced his entrance.

Instead, he was sneaking in quietly closing the door behind him. He walked over to the bed and whispered, "Wake up Little Darling. Time to get up and give your old Fred a kiss." He leaned his entire body over the bed and gave me a kiss I was sure would bruise my lips. I still pretended to be asleep.

He yanked back the sheet. I could feel the morning breeze on my skin. I was well aware my baby doll nightgown covered very little. I also could feel his eyes taking every inch of the picture in front of him.

He rubbed my bare leg and said, "Come on, now. I know you're awake. You can't fool me."

I couldn't have responded even if I wanted to. I was paralyzed just like the time my Grandma and I saw a copperhead snake on the trail down by the creek. She told me to stand still and not move.

I was well aware there was danger staring right at me, but I did not want to give him the satisfaction of seeing me see him.

I was well aware there was danger staring right at me.

Instead, I kept my eyes closed, held my breath and prayed over and over again in my mind. "Help me, Jesus. Help me, Jesus."

Every second of the next few minutes became etched in my memory. His hands moved from my legs to places I knew Mom would be angry I had allowed him to touch. What could I do? He was a grown man. I was just a fly on the wall compared to him. I wanted to scream as his hands lifted my nightgown to my chin and began exploring every inch of my body.

The touching became groping. It hurt my body and my soul. Frozen in time and space, my mind went numb; my body went limp. I wanted to be anywhere but there.

I tried to go elsewhere in my mind and think good thoughts, but I could only think of how I could get away from him. I was so afraid of what he would do. He stopped for a moment and I heard him take off his shirt and then fiddle with something, maybe a zipper. After a cuss word left his lips, he continued his exploration. It felt like my mind left my body.

I tried to go elsewhere in my mind and think good thoughts.

He jerked me like he was trying to wake me up. When I refused to open my eyes, he said in a hoarse whisper. "I said open your eyes or else." What else could be worse than this? I tried again to pray silently and urgently, "Help, God. Help!"

He was still there, and I wasn't sure I could endure anything else. I thought about what I could do to stop him. I could claw his face. I could kick him in just the right place. I could scream at the top of my lungs. I saw every action in my mind, but I could not make my body move.

Then, I heard my answer to prayer. "Fred, time for breakfast." It was Minnie calling from the bottom of the stairs just outside the room we were in.

"Be right there, Sugar," Fred answered. I could hear him moving and grabbing his shirt from where he had thrown it on the floor. He leaned down close to me and said gruffly in my ear, "Open your eyes."

I disobeyed. I couldn't move. I waited until I heard the door close. Even then, it was several more minutes before I could allow myself to open my eyes. The fear of him was still very alive in me. I didn't know if he would eat his breakfast quickly and come back or not. It motivated me to get up, grab some clothes and run downstairs to the bathroom. I could hear laughter coming from the kitchen, so I knew he was entertaining everyone there.

I locked the bathroom door and took a quick bath. I wanted to wash him off of me. I had no idea it would be years before that would happen. It wouldn't be me who set me free from those memories. It would be the God who heard me and answered my prayer that day.

SELF-PROTECTING

Although I wanted to tell Grandma what happened, I couldn't. Minnie was her best friend. What if Grandma didn't believe me? What if she thought it was all my fault? Was it all my fault? I didn't know for sure.

Fred went to church every Sunday. He was supposed to be a good, upstanding man. Maybe it was my fault because Dad always told me not to wear shorts or sleeveless tops. It was summer. I had worn both. Maybe I enticed him?

I couldn't tell Dad. He'd think it was my fault. I couldn't tell Mom. She had enough problems dealing with everything she was going through. I decided I would have to protect myself. First, I wouldn't stay at Grandma's while Minnie and Fred were there. If I had to go to an event where he was, I would plan to be where he wasn't. I would stay far away even if it meant I had to be rude.

Hiding the truth was harder than I thought it would be. There were times Mom made me kiss Fred even though I refused. I allowed it but pulled away quickly. Fred gave me a look which made me want to scream. I prayed he wouldn't ever come back to visit.

> Hiding the truth was harder than I thought it would be.

If he did, it was when I was older and was able to make excuses to stay away. Carrying the weight of what happened was overwhelming to me. I told no one until Roy and I decided to get married when I was 23. I only told him because I didn't know how the Fred issue would affect intimacy.

I had steered clear of most boys. Part of this was because of Fred, the other part was because of a boy my parents let me date when I was only 12. This was too close to the Fred incident, but of course, they didn't know that.

Tim[3] was a good church-going boy who was not old enough to drive. This was probably the only reason Mom let me go out with him at such a young age. She seemed to think cars were the only places girls could get into compromising conditions.

Tim was a gentleman, though. We only had three or four dates that summer but being so young and naive I was head over heels in love with him. I just knew one day we would get married probably before finishing high school. He had said nothing to make me think that. It was just my imagination, running 10,000 steps ahead.

When school started, I went to junior high while he went to high school. It wasn't a month into school before he brought his new high school girlfriend to church with him. I thought he was still my boyfriend. After school started, he hadn't called or asked me out. I didn't know how these things worked. I'd never had a real boyfriend before. It wasn't his fault that he broke my heart. I had allowed myself to fall in love with him.

Once again, I decided to self-protect. I promised myself I would never fall in love again. It hurt too much. I kept this promise for a long time. I dated a few young men, but none tugged at my heart until I met a tall, lanky blonde guy named Roy at the New Wine Coffeehouse in the summer of 1973.

We've been married since 1977, so I think it has worked out. Before we got married, I told him about the Fred incident. He listened, held me close and told me he would protect me. That was all I needed to hear. It was a perfect solution whenever he was with me, but he couldn't be with me all the time. When he wasn't there, the fear would come back.

FAT SHAMING

About two years after we got married, I was working for a denominational headquarters. My boss had told me during a performance review he loved my work. He should. I was working 60 hours a week for a 40-hour-week salaried job. However, he said I should lose weight and get nicer clothes.

I was angry. We would call this fat-shaming today. I probably weighed about 260 pounds at this time. I needed to lose 100 pounds. At first, I rebelled against what he said. Then, I noticed my pastor's wife had lost a lot of weight. She and I talked, and she told me the name of the program she was on, promised to pray with me and be a buddy on my journey.

I justified putting the expensive diet program on a credit card because it would be saving my job. It took a lot of hard work and about nine months, but I did it. I had weighed by my scales and had reached the magic number, but I wanted to go to the program's office to officially weigh. At lunch, I went and weighed and sure enough. I had done it. I had lost 100 pounds. I drove back to the office on cloud nine.

Extra pounds can be my protection against the unwanted advances of men.

I walked into the building and got on the elevator with one of the department directors. I knew his name, but he traveled a lot and I hadn't dealt with him much. When the elevators closed, he looked me up and down and said, "You're looking really good today."

I was immediately back on the trail and a copperhead snake was staring me in the face. I froze. I didn't know what to say. He kept talking and said something like, "We'll have to get together sometime."

As soon as the elevator doors opened, I ran to my office. I had interpreted his actions as an older man coming on to me, much like Fred. I realized my fear of certain types of men was still very much alive.

I didn't see this as a stronghold then. I should have because that day I made a willful plan to start eating sugar again. I went downstairs on break and bought two candy bars and a diet soda. I hadn't had either of those in over nine months, but it didn't matter. I had to protect myself.

If I hadn't lost 100 pounds, the department director wouldn't have come on to me. If I didn't look good, I wouldn't have enticed him. Extra pounds can be my protection against the men who are like copperhead snakes in this world. It's a way to protect myself.

This stronghold of fear became entrenched in me. I knew it was crazy. The department director probably wasn't coming on to me, I just thought he was. The 11-year-old me who was molested still believed I was in danger.

FORGIVENESS

I didn't understand how I could be an intelligent adult woman and still believe this lie, but I did. It was such a stronghold even when I forgave Fred during a Joyce Meyer conference, it did not erase my need to self-protect.

Forgiving Fred, though, was a first step in breaking the stronghold of I need to protect myself. Whenever I would think about Fred, I would see him as a huge monster in my mind and I was a teeny, tiny wimp. When I forgave him, I saw him as a shriveled up little old man compared to me. I could take him on easily.

When I forgave Fred, I was a super morbidly obese woman. I saw him as a shrimp compared to me. On some level, I thought my self-protection of making myself bigger was working. God had torn down my fear of men, but the other stronghold of I have to self-protect was still there.

A few years later, I went through a course called Family of Origin with Russ as the leader. A woman who was a sexual abuse counselor was also taking the course. When I presented my family of origin, I talked about the molestation with Fred. Russ asked the counselor a question mainly so I'd hear the answer.

"What do you call a man who sexually abuses children?" he asked.

"A pedophile," she answered.

"Does a pedophile just have one victim?"

"No, he has multiple victims."

"Does he grab them off the street or how does he find his victims?"

"Most of the time pedophiles are very good at grooming victims, which means they entice them with candy or gifts. They are usually outgoing people everyone loves, and no one would suspect what they are doing."

It was my turn, "So they might give kids money?"

"Oh yes," she said. "Especially if the kids are motivated by money. They are good at reading what kids want."

"How many kids might they abuse?" I asked.

"As many as they can," she answered.

"So, it wasn't my fault?"

"It wasn't your fault." This time they answered in unison.

I felt so good I could have cried. Knowing it wasn't my fault was what I needed to know.

KNOWLEDGE HELPS

When we are children, we make decisions based on what we know at the time. When I was 11, I knew nothing about what Fred's problem was. I was an adult with children of my own before I discovered what pedophile even means.

Since then, I've gone through training for dealing with mentally challenged individuals who are sexual predators. Those I've worked with who have mental challenges can conduct themselves in a normal fashion if they know they have oversight of a caregiver who knows their problems and their boundaries.

In situations where individuals are of normal intelligence and have this problem, they are not usually overt about it. They aren't likely to lure a child away without first knowing the child will go with them willingly or at least won't tell anyone. I see how this played out with Fred.

He planned his adventure with me. He groomed me and chose me because he knew my home situation. I also happened to be in his target age range. Knowing this helped me understand the situation a lot better.

GOD IS MY PROTECTOR

This was the logical truth I needed. I also needed to embrace the spiritual truth God is with me. Understanding this began to release more freedom into my life.[4] Jesus had already set me free. I had to learn how to live in my new-found freedom. Self-protection was no longer necessary. God had removed my need to constantly be on guard. I finally began to trust Him to protect me.

When I began to look for them, I found many promises that reinforced my understanding of God is my protector. Probably the most helpful chapter and the one I return to time and time again is Psalm 91.

"He will cover you with his feathers. He will shelter you with His wings. His faithful promises are your armor and protection. Do not be afraid of the terrors of the night, nor the arrow that flies in the day. Do not dread the disease that stalks in darkness, nor the disaster that strikes at midday."[5]

"If you make the Lord your refuge, if you make the Most High your shelter, no evil will conquer you; no plague will come near your home. For He will order His angels to protect you wherever you go. They will hold you up with their hands so you won't even hurt your foot on a stone."[6]

Not living in fear is the best feeling in the world.

How could I be afraid when I have a faithful God who protects me with His promises and sends His angels to take care of me? These days I am constantly aware of God's presence with me in the form of the Holy Spirit, but I have also been aware many times of His angels protecting me, especially one time when my little Honda Fit bounced off of a semi twice on the interstate. The car was totaled. I only had a bruise where the seat belt went across my shoulder.

When I finally pulled over to the side of the road, my first words were, "God, you must still have something left for me to do here on earth because I should be dead right now." Roy took me to see the car once it had been towed to the junkyard. The major dents were on the driver's side. One was behind the driver's door. The other was in front of it. The only place without a massive hit was the driver's door where I was sitting. My angel had been standing right there protecting me.

ENDNOTES

1. Not his real name.
2. Not her real name.
3. Not his real name
4. John 8:32 TPT
5. Psalm 91:4-6 NLT
6. Psalm 91:9-12 NLT

CHAPTER 7

I MATTER TO GOD

Mom always described herself as being "nervous." From listening in on other adults discussing her situation, I heard the words manic depression, anxiety and agoraphobia used to describe her, but all I knew was if she was sick, I had to fix supper. If we didn't have clothes to wear to school, I needed to do a load of laundry and I had to make sure my brother and sister were somewhere near the house. If the house was a mess, I needed to clean it up.

When Mom wasn't feeling well, as the oldest I had a lot of responsibilities. I was needed and felt it. Dad regularly told me this, as did my grandparents. I heard it from every place except the one place which really mattered. I never heard it from Mom.

There was a tension between us that seemed to never go away. It seems like it was always there. It made me feel even though I was working hard to help her, I didn't matter to her.

We lived in a small 800-square foot house with three small bedrooms. My sister and I had a room with bunk beds which was more like the end of a hallway. My brother slept in a converted back porch and my parents in a walled-off end of the living room. To escape her moods, there was no place to go except outside or up to the attic.

Mom rarely went up to the attic, so this was where I cleared out a space of my own. An old mattress and a few quilts and I had a place to get away from the world. It didn't matter if it was hot in the summer and cold in the winter, it was my place to find peace and hear myself think.

I looked forward to the days she sat in her chair in the living room staring into space or lost in a book. Those days she was quiet. I would do what needed to be done, then do my homework and everything went fine. On other days, though, I couldn't do anything right. Everything I did made her mad.

I CAN'T WIN FOR LOSING

On her angry days, she seemed to pick fights with me just because. The one I remember vividly happened when I was home from college for Christmas break. I already had a job lined up which I went to the next day. I came in from working and could immediately tell Mom was mad at me. I hadn't even been there two days and somehow, I had already made her angry.

She had gotten a letter in the mail saying the balance on my college tuition was due and if it wasn't paid, I wouldn't be able to go back to school and finish my senior year. My parents hadn't been able to pay it in September. Had I known this earlier, I would have worked more hours while at school.

"You are the reason we have no money," she screamed in my face. "If we weren't spending everything for your college and sending you money every month for food, I could buy a new dress every now and then. You are an ungrateful child."

"I will quit school then," I said. "I'll work more, save money and finish next year or when I can."

"Oh yeah, so then everyone will think we are horrible parents for making you quit the last semester of college."

"Mom, you said you don't have the money. I'll figure it out. I'll put in more hours at my job. I'll see if they'll give me an extension, a payment plan or a student loan."

"Oh, no you don't. You really know how to rub it in, don't you? You won't make me into the bad guy. You are going back even if we have to eat beans and rice for a year."

Somewhere during this conversation, she got so angry she threatened to spank me with a belt. I grabbed her arm and said, "No, you won't. I'm an adult now." Then like a scared rabbit, I ran to the attic, fell on the old mattress, burrowed under my quilt and blubbered like a baby for hours. Tears wash the soul, but they didn't help this time. I couldn't win for losing. There was no good way out of the situation.

Tears wash the soul, but they didn't help this time.

As far back as I can remember Mom and I would have these kinds of no-win arguments. If I argued with her, she would flip-flop on me and say something different. It didn't matter because in the end whatever I said was always wrong.

What I felt didn't matter to her and the more I told myself this, the more I believed she disapproved of everything about me. I couldn't do anything right. Why is it we always want approval from the one person in the world who never seems to give it to us? I just couldn't win for losing with her and yet, if I said nothing then she would take it to mean I believed whatever outrageous thing she was either accusing me of or trying to argue with me about.

MOTHER-DAUGHTER TEA

Mom didn't come to any of my school events. She never met any of my teachers. She didn't go to plays or concerts. She didn't go to parent-teacher conferences. When I told her I was going to join Brownies in second grade, she found me a second-hand Brownie dress and beanie. This was one of the best things she ever did for me.

So when my troop held the first mother-daughter tea I was sure she would come. I told her about the tea weeks before and even put it on her calendar. I asked her if she would come and she said, "We'll see." I took this to mean she would. I was only eight. So far, she hadn't disappointed me too badly. I believed she would come.

The morning of the tea I got dressed in my Brownie dress and beanie and reminded her she needed to come inside after school instead of picking me up.

"Why?" she said.

"Remember it's the Brownie Mother-Daughter Tea. All the girls have to bring their moms. You'll be there, right?"

"We'll see."

"I'll wait for you right beside the front door," I said as I ran out the door to walk to school.

I was so excited to share the tea with Mom that I could barely focus in class. After class, I waited by the door. I saw all the mothers come in, join their daughters and walk down the hall to the cafeteria.

When no one was left, I got the message. Mom was sick again. She wasn't coming. I felt the tears beginning, ran to the restroom and got in a stall before anyone saw me crying. If I mattered to Mom, she would be here. She had to know how much this meant to me. Yet, even at eight, I had begun to realize my feelings didn't matter. The only emotions at play were hers. They ran the show.

While I was in the bathroom drowning my sorrows in my tears, Mrs. Rice came in to clean. She and her husband were the school janitors. She asked, "Is anyone in here?" I said I was. She asked if I was finished and could come out because she needed to mop the floors.

When I exited the stall, she said, "Wait. What's the matter?"

The waterworks let go again and I told her how Mom didn't care about me because she hadn't come to the tea and now, I couldn't go because I didn't have a mother.

I told her how Mom didn't care about me.

Mrs. Rice listened and then, ran water over a paper towel and told me to come and wash my face. "I'm sure your mother would be here if she could," she said as she helped me.

"No," I said. "She can't. She's sick."

"Tell you what," she said. "How about I come and be your stand-in mother?"

"You'd do that for me?" I asked.

"Sure, I've done it for several girls over the years. I kind of like it."

I grinned from ear to ear as she walked down to the cafeteria with me. I thought a few of the girls were jealous because Mrs. Rice was my stand-in mother. Everyone loved Mrs. Rice.

As soon as refreshments were served, she had to leave. She whispered in my ear, "Thank you for letting me be your mother for the afternoon. I'd be happy to do it again."

What started as a horrible, no good, very bad day ended well because of a hard-working woman, who probably had to put in some extra time because of the time she took off for me. I mattered to Mrs. Rice.

When the mother-daughter banquet at my church I was attending came around I didn't even ask Mom. I asked the church organist, Mrs. Brown. She didn't have any children and was happy to accompany me to the banquet.

Mrs. Brown was a great stand-in mom. It made me feel good to have someone at my church who cared about me. For years I gave Mrs. Brown a card every Mother's Day and always got her a corsage for the banquet.

Thank God for the Mrs. Rices and Mrs. Browns in the world. I mattered to them, but it didn't make up for the fact I felt didn't matter to the woman who gave me birth.

DISMANTLING THE LIE

The lie I don't matter to Mom became a stronghold because I allowed it to grow every year. I didn't know how to deal with the feeling that I was an orphan even though I had a mother.

Mom's treatment of me always made me cry from the eight-year-old incident up to the 20-year-old incident. I didn't like crying. I felt like crying was for wimps and people who were crazy, like Mom. She was making me feel crazy.

The only time I felt like I could deal with the way she treated me was to retreat to Grandma's on the weekend. At Grandma's all my cares and worries and concerns seemed to fade away. She talked to me like a real person. She regularly gave me hugs and told me she loved me. The stronghold of I don't matter to Mom was still there, but it was just drowned out by a growing dependence I was developing on comfort foods.

I had not dealt with the lie that had become a stronghold. I had only shelved it thinking that was when I was a kid.

Even after I was married and had children, I had not dealt with the lie which had now become a stronghold. I had simply shelved it thinking that was when I was a kid. Mom was sick so I can't blame her for what she did. I'm an adult now. She's changed. We'll let bygones be bygones.

All this time I was gaining weight. I felt like I needed to talk to someone because even though I knew how to lose weight but my body refused to cooperate. There was a counselor who worked at the clinic I went to, so I decided to go see her. It was covered by insurance and I figured why not? It might help.

On my first visit, I told the counselor why I was there. I said nothing about Mom, but the first thing she said was, "Tell me about your mother." I thought, what does my mother have to do with my weight gain? Still, I shared about Mom's manic depression, wide mood swings, anger outbursts, lack of involvement in my school life, never coming to my events and how I didn't matter to her.

When I was finished, she said, "How do you feel towards your mother?"

I said, "She couldn't help it. She was sick. She didn't know what she was doing."

THE CHALLENGE

The counselor challenged me saying I must have some deeper feelings regarding how she treated me. The more she prodded me to reveal my anger towards her, I couldn't. All I could hear was Dad saying, "We need to pray for your mom. She's sick. She doesn't know what she's doing."

At the end of the session, she told me to write two letters to Mom about how I feel. She wanted me to start each letter with, "I'm angry because," and then fill in what I was angry about. I was to use my right hand to write the letter from my adult point of view. Then, I was to write another letter using my left hand and write it from the point of view of me as an eight-year-old.

I was skeptical of anything coming of this, but when I did it, I couldn't believe what happened. The adult me wrote a letter that included all the reasons why I couldn't be angry with Mom like her being a loving grandmother. There was a night and day difference between the adult me writing to Mom and the eight-year-old me writing to Mommy.

DEAR MOMMY,

I'm angry because you are treating me like a child when I've had to be the adult all this time.

I'm angry because you leave us sometimes to go to the hospital to get better, but you don't get better.

I'm angry because you never come to any of my assemblies, plays or other school events.

I'm angry because you never come to my mother-daughter teas or banquets.

I'm angry because you never come to my parent-teacher conferences.

I'm angry because you never compliment me on my grades.

I'm angry because I can't bring any of my friends' home because I never know what kind of mood, you'll be in.

I'm angry because you scream at me for ridiculous things which make no sense.

I'm angry because you spank me in anger.

I'm angry because I feel like I don't love you and yet, I love you so much it hurts my tummy.

I'm angry because you are not the kind of mother, I want you to be.

I'm angry because I have to do stuff I don't know how to do.

I'm angry because you're supposed to be my mom, but I feel like I'm raising you!

Teresa, Age 8

As I reread what I'd written I was shocked. I didn't know I had all those feelings. I didn't like the anger rising in me. On the other hand, it was intensely freeing. I no longer had to keep my emotions hidden in the back closet. I could own my anger. It could become part of who I was.

I didn't know it at the time, but this was the first step to breaking the stronghold I had constructed. What I had to do was understand how the whole scenario had played out in me as a child. I had to understand my anger towards Mom was real.

The first step towards forgiving anyone is to recognize they have done something which has made us angry. If we pretend we aren't angry about what happened, it only allows us to construct the stronghold more securely so no truth will permeate it. This means it will become an even bigger problem. For me, it became I don't matter to Mom, but I'm not angry about it because she was sick. I'm doing just fine eating everything I want to make the pain go away.

> If we pretend we aren't angry about what happened, it only allows us to construct the stronghold more securely so no truth will permeate it.

I hadn't dealt with the real issue which was that I was angry and needed to forgive Mom. By this time, she had already moved to heaven. I used the letter I wrote as the little girl me to forgive her for each thing on the list.

After Mom passed away, we were cleaning out drawers in the buffet she had in the dining room. I knew she kept newspaper clippings in one of the drawers, but I didn't know what was in the cabinet beneath it. When we opened the door out fell every article I had ever written for organizations, magazines and newspapers I had worked for.

I was flabbergasted. Mom never complimented me on anything I wrote. I didn't even know she knew about many of those articles. I asked Dad how she got them because I knew I hadn't sent them to her. He said he didn't know. She hadn't even shown them to him.

> The truth hit me like a lightning bolt. I did matter to Mom.

Then the truth hit me like a lightning bolt. I did matter to Mom. She was proud of me. She did love me. She had been collecting articles from the time I started my career. She knew I had a gift. She just was silently supporting me.

When I realized this, it broke something else loose inside me. I know a mother's role involves comfort and teaching her children. If our mothers have filled those roles well, we can better accept the role of the Holy Spirit as one who comforts and guides us. Mom didn't fill those roles well for me. She was absent even though she was there. This was the opposite of comfort. It was confusion and lack of peace or comfort.

Even though Grandma comforted me, there was still the absence of a mother and I felt it even as an adult. Understanding I did matter to her helped me to begin to accept the role of the Holy Spirit in my life. I saw Him as a confusing whirlwind of colors, sounds and movements. It was the same picture I had of Mom.

Knowing I mattered to her helped me understand that I matter to the Holy Spirit as well. Knowing this helped me accept the comfort of the Holy Spirit. For too long when I thought of comfort, I thought of food because that was one of Grandma's ways of comforting me. Now I had a different way to look at comfort. It is the abiding presence of the love, peace and power of the Holy Spirit leading me forward.

I MATTER TO GOD

The realization hit me strongly. I matter to God. If I were the only person in the world, He still would have sent His Son to die for me. It's hard to explain how uncovering all the stories I'd written that Mom had saved made me understand the truth I did matter, not just to her, but also to God.

His hand was all over finding those articles and the fact I was there when it happened. It still mystifies me as to how she got all of them in the first place. God knew the day I discovered those articles would help cement in my heart that I do matter.

He was looking out for me throughout my entire life. Even if I never mattered to Mom, I know I matter to God. His constant presence with me every minute of every day. Even while I was still rebelling against God, Christ died for me.[1] There is no greater love than this. That alone should tell me I matter to God.

It's a given in this world I will have trouble, but I can keep going forward because Jesus overcame the world.[2] He will help me do the same. He is a gentleman who wants to carry my burdens, worries and concerns because He really does care for me.[3]

When I am tempted to go against what I know He wants for me, He shows me how to do the right thing.[4] He provides a way out. I just need to take it. He is with me wherever I go.[5] He strengthens and helps me.[6] He meets all my needs.[7] He is my refuge and my shield.[8] He guides me to the right path.[9] He tells me when I stray off His path and points me in the way I should go.[10]

"The Lord your God is in your midst, a warrior who saves. He will rejoice over you with joy; He will be quiet in His love, He will rejoice over you with shouts of joy."[11]

I matter to God. We all do.

ENDNOTES

1. Romans 5:8 NIV
2. John 16:33 NIV
3. 2 Peter 5:7 NIV
4. 1 Cor. 10:13 NIV
5. Joshua 1:9 NIV
6. Isaiah 41:10 NIV
7. Philippians 4:19 NIV
8. Psalm 119:114 NIV
9. Psalm 23:3 NIV
10. Isaiah 30:21 NIV
11. Zephaniah 3:17 AMP

"Have I not commanded you? Be strong and courageous. Do not be afraid; do not be discouraged, for the Lord your God will be with you wherever you go."

JOSHUA 1:9 NIV

CHAPTER 10

GOD VALUES ME

I was in eighth grade when Mrs. Grabner, the sponsor for our junior high newspaper, made me the fiction editor. It was an honor because editorial positions usually only went to ninth graders. As a seventh-grader, I had written poems and short stories that had been published.

It wasn't editor-in-chief, and it wasn't the news editor or editorial editor, but still, it felt good to be noticed. Mrs. Grabner told me she saw promise in my writing. Her words were encouraging.

It felt good to be noticed.

To say it gave me a big head was an understatement. I loved being acknowledged. I ate up encouragement like it was going out of style. My love language is words of affirmation. It makes a lot of sense with what happened next and why it affected me so profoundly. I love positive words, but negative words always feel like a slap in the face.

PROFOUND DISCOURAGEMENT

"Mrs. Grabner made me fiction editor of the newspaper today," I said at the supper table.

"That's wonderful," Dad said tousling my hair.

"Yeah, and I think when I go to college, I'm going to major in creative writing so I can learn how to be an author and write novels."

Mom looked over her glasses at me and said, "When you go to college, you will major in something practical so you can get a paying job when you graduate."

"Authors get paid," I said.

"Writing a book is difficult. It's more than knowing how to write. It's having the right story which really makes a difference." Mom wouldn't back down, but then I was just as stubborn.

"I love stories. I love writing stories. It's what I want to do," I said firmly in my eighth-grade, all-knowing sort of way.

"Only if you can get a teaching certificate to go with it. Then at least you can get a job while you do your writing hobby."

"I don't want to be a teacher. Maybe I'll marry a rich guy."

"Good luck with that," she said casting a sideways glance at Dad. There was always a bit of tension between them about money.

She continued, "Even if you could write a novel, there's getting a publisher to publish it and then, people to buy it. Then authors have to sell a lot of books to make any money at all. They only make a very small percentage of the price of a book."

"Don't you think I'm a good writer, Mom?" I shouldn't have asked. I should have let it go. I should have, but I didn't. When I heard her next words, they hit hard.

"Teresa, you will never make money by writing a book. Just forget about it and focus on something else."

That was it. My dreams of being a fiction author were not just dashed, but crushed, demolished, obliterated completely with those few words. "You'll never make money writing a book."

Because Mom gave me a dose of truth, I focused on finding another way to make my mark writing. I knew from early on writing was a gift God had given me. I was surprised to learn there weren't very many of my classmates who loved essay questions. I could always ace an essay question even if I didn't know much about the subject.

In my sophomore year in high school, I took a journalism class and just before my junior year I was named editorial editor. It was also the year my favorite journalism teacher quit. In her place came a teacher who had graduated from a Christian university. It was the only year she taught at our school and I know she was there just for me. She recommended me for a journalism scholarship to the college she graduated from and told me about other scholarships which made it possible for me to attend there.

BECOMING AN AUTHOR

The crushing blow Mom dealt me regarding never being able to make money writing books followed me through the decades. I did not write a book until 2013. It wasn't a fiction book. It was nonfiction, as have been the others I've written since.

She was wrong in saying I couldn't make money writing books because I have made money as an author, although not as a fiction author yet. Part of being able to make a bit of money as an author has been because of technological changes that have come about with book publishing since the 1960s when Mom was giving me her advice. I can now self-publish my own books, something she never foresaw.

For many years, I held a grievance against Mom for those discouraging words. I felt if she hadn't discouraged me maybe I could have been a great fiction writer. I see this is not the truth. She was giving me advice based on how publishing operated back then. What she said was true for that time. I would have had to have a novel written, get the attention of an agent and have a publisher. Unknown authors weren't just discovered from the pages of self-published books like some have been in this day and age.

She did give me good advice even though I didn't like it. By steering me away from fiction writing, I chose the path of telling the truth through journalistic stories. I became good at it. It's something I can do in my sleep. I place a high value on honesty, so I've long since forgiven her for being honest with me. I've even asked God to forgive me for holding a grudge against her for so long and blaming my lack of becoming an author on her.

WHO AM I?

There is one big issue in all of this, though. Ever since I can remember I felt like I needed to know what I was going to be when I grew up. When I was a kid, I had many great grandparents and grandparents alive along with a wide variety of aunts, uncles, great aunts and uncles, even a few great-great aunts.

They all would ask me, "What are you going to be when you grow up?" It seemed like a question I should know the answer to. It was a life-defining question. What I thought they meant was, what job are you going to pursue as a career?

Some of the other girls would answer, "I want to be a mommy." That's all they wanted. I wanted to be a mom, but I also wanted to work too. I was wired to be a doer. Doing things defined me.

When I took the Enneagram test, I wasn't surprised to find out I am a three, which is an achiever or in other words, a doer. As an achiever, I want to be successful in whatever I do. I want what I do to be valuable. I don't want to be seen as incompetent, inefficient or worthless.

All my life, I've sought to show my value by what I do and how I succeed.

All my life, I've sought to show my value by what I do and how I succeed. It started in elementary school when my second-grade teacher, Mrs. Cornelison gave me all E's on my report card the last day of school.

She told me I could be anything I wanted to be if I studied hard. So, I studied. At first, I did it so I could return at the end of each year and show her my report card. Then, it became a game I played with myself. I didn't do it to learn anything. I did it to get a good grade. Good grades made me feel I had achieved something. Plus, Grandma gave me a dollar for every E on my report card. I finally had value.

Achievement and performance felt tied to who I was. Without my college degree in journalism, who was I? Without my job experience with several denominational headquarters, organizations and newspapers, who was I?

If someone asked me who I was, I would answer with whatever job I had at the time. It defined who I was. After we had two children, I quit my full-time job to edit and publish a regional Christian newspaper. It made no money, but it was what God told me I would be doing one day.

I was in junior high when I read the book, *In His Steps* and I felt like God spoke to me. He said, "One day you will edit and publish a Christian newspaper solely financed by commercial ad revenue." I asked Dad if there were any newspapers like this. He said the only Christian newspapers being published then were financed by denominations.

I hadn't had many spiritual experiences, but I knew I had heard from God and one day this would happen. It was the reason I got a degree in journalism and religion. Even when I graduated from college in 1975, I knew of no such newspapers.

ONE DREAM COME TRUE

It was in 1989 when I was working for a local hospital, I met a man who was an ad rep for a local Christian radio station. I was the volunteer public relations director for a large church. He would stop by my office at the hospital to pick up ads for the church.

One day, he told me it was the last day he'd be calling on me. He was leaving the station to start a regional Christian newspaper solely supported by advertising revenue. My mouth fell open. He was describing exactly what God told me I would be doing.

At first, I was mad at God. I wanted this to be my achievement. Then I realized God was giving me an opportunity to learn everything I could about publishing. In talking to me about it, the new publisher asked if I'd like to help. I knew he wasn't a writer. He was a salesman. He needed me.

I agreed to attend the meeting he'd set up with another one of his friends. The next week I met Linda, who happened to have three boys, the oldest of whom was the same age as my son. She was a photographer and writer and had done a church newspaper, so she knew the business.

We helped him put together three editions before he realized he couldn't make a living doing it. He found a job as a journalist for a Christian organization on the east coast. He gave the publication to us.

GOOD NEWS

This consisted of the name, which we changed to *Good News Journal* and a very short list of advertisers. To pay the newspaper's printing and distribution bills we needed more advertisers. To get advertisers we needed to guarantee them a bigger circulation.

It was Linda's idea to insert the paper in our local newspaper just like any other advertising flier. Back then they would let us do this even though we also had ads in our publication.

Doing this meant we immediately got enough advertising support to afford to print the paper and insert it. We also delivered to churches and businesses in a wide area of

Missouri. Our circulation grew to 100,000. I made no money doing this, but I loved it. I felt I had found the reason I was put on this earth.

Around 2000 I also began publishing *Family Magazine,* which was a Christian parenting magazine my kids and I delivered to churches and schools in our area and surrounding towns. Writing, editing and publishing became my identity. It was who I was. Then the internet began to explode, and free newspaper publications went by the wayside. By 2002 we had ceased publishing *Good News Journal.* By 2008, I had stopped publishing *Family Magazine* and the bottom fell out of my world.

WHO AM I NOW?

My reaction to what was happening hit me hard. I felt extreme sadness. I had been put out to pasture by God even though I was still in my 50s. I was angry that my job, and therefore my identity, had been ripped from me.

Even though I tried to find someone to blame, but it seemed the only one I could really blame was God. My thoughts and feelings told me I wasn't fulfilling the purpose He had for me. I wasn't valuable to God.

"Why would You give me this great job only to snatch it from me?" I screamed at Him. When I wasn't mad at God, I sat and moped and continued to gain weight. Without the publications to write, edit, publish and deliver who was I? Eating had already become my way of coping with feelings I didn't like. Now it felt like my life was over and food was the only thing I could count on.

It's not like I was doing nothing. In 1998 we had started providing care for a mentally challenged foster son. I had plenty of work to do managing his needs, plus those of my two children. We had done this to help with our monetary issue and because we felt like we had something to offer him. It didn't help at all with my identity issue.

I was a foster mom and although it involved a lot of work, it didn't fit my vocational calling. However, if I was contributing to the family income, I could keep writing, editing and publishing the newspapers while still being at home.

> I was consumed by a stronghold of performance.

With the publications gone, all of the things I identified with as my purpose were gone, and I was left feeling empty. Despite having a full life, I felt useless because I had put faith in my ability to write, edit and publish. I'm a writer. Writers write. When I wasn't writing, who was I? I was sad and depressed. I was a big, fat blob sitting at home eating candy all day.

I had constructed the lie I am only valuable when I am publishing something. I was consumed by a stronghold of performance I didn't even realize had taken me captive. I was turning to food to relieve my lack of value and worth.

I AM MORE THAN WHAT I DO

"I am more than what I do," Paula Faris, the author of *Called Out*, said recently. "Freedom is knowing who I am outside of what I do." This truth was exactly what I needed to hear back in 2008. Sadly, I didn't hear then. I wallowed in despair for five years but also threw myself into the weight loss journey I knew God had for me. It was 2013 when He tapped me on the shoulder and asked me to write a book about losing 250 pounds. I should have been elated. Instead, I was scared. Could I do this? I'd been working on my weight and not doing a lot of writing.

We were still managing mentally challenged foster adults in our home. I wasn't looking for another way to make money, but I did want to do what God wanted me to do. By October 2013 the book was written and on Amazon. By January of 2014, the book became number one in Christian weight loss memoirs on Amazon.

Finally, I felt I had value again. When the book became number one on Amazon in its category my life got really busy. I hired a full-time house manager to take care of the clients we had. When someone asks me who I am, I know they want to know what I do. For those in-between years, I would say I managed a home for mentally challenged young adults. After I wrote *Sweet Grace* when they'd ask, I would say, I am an author, coach and speaker. Every time I said those words, they made me feel valuable because of what I did.

GOD CALLED ME OUT

Hearing Faris' words went straight to my heart when I heard them. It reminded me of the stronghold I had addressed years ago, but I knew there was still more work I needed to do in this area. God told me I was still living inside a lie. He said, "You are still believing your value is in what you do instead of who you are."

He was telling me I needed to know who I am without my job. I do know who I am. I am a whole, healthy, happy woman. I know this as a truth, but the problem is I regularly feel if I am not doing something in my chosen vocational field it doesn't matter who I am. I still believed if I was doing nothing then I wasn't worth anything to God. Therefore, my value is not in who I am. It is in what I do.

On the days I relax and take some time off, I tend to feel like I am worthless. God wants me to see I am just as valuable, if not more valuable to Him then than when I am working. When I'm working hard it can be like trying to push a huge boulder up a hill. I don't feel God's presence when I'm pushing hard to meet a self-imposed deadline. I'm learning that when I take time to unplug from electronics, relax, empty my mind of my to-do list and am simply available to God, He always speaks to me.

It has been hard for me to understand that God belives I am enough just like I am.

I had been begging God to give me the title for this book for months. It was only when I decided to take a drive through the country God saw fit to drop the title into my mind. I wasn't asking Him for it. I wasn't thinking about it. The car was quiet, and my mind was unencumbered. This is an environment that invites God to speak. It's always when I can listen without other interruptions.

It has been hard for me to understand that God believes I am enough just like I am. He's watched me from the day I was born. He created me in His image and knows everything about me.[1] He knew what I would do and when I would do it. Nothing about me has taken Him by surprise.

"It's in Christ that we find out who we are and what we are living for. Long before we first heard of Christ and got our hopes up, He had His eye on us, had designs on us for glorious living, part of the overall purpose He is working out in everything and everyone."[2]

I was created on purpose for a purpose. I have value because God made me. I don't have to do anything to prove to Him. I just have to be who He created me to be. He and He alone has planned my future.

I was created on purpose for a purpose. I have value because God made me.

God has a destiny and a purpose for me. He has given me gifts, talents and abilities. I don't need to be concerned about how He is going to utilize those. All I have to be concerned about is loving and following Him. If I am doing that He will work everything out to fulfill the purpose He has for me. Nothing I can do will hurry it up or change it. I just need to trust Him. I just need to follow Him.

The stronghold of I have to do more to have value to God is broken in Jesus' name because I know the truth. I am already enough in Him. I don't have to achieve anything to earn His grace. I already have it.

I don't have to do anything, but love God to be valuable to Him. I choose to be available to Him for whatever He has for me. I never want to be too busy to stop and commune with Him. I can do that and be even more valuable than when I am working myself to death.

It's time to get quiet in His presence. It's time to love Him by honoring Him with my undivided attention. It's in this place I know I am valuable to God just because I'm me.

ENDNOTES

1. Psalm 139:13-16 NLT
2. Ephesians 1:11-12 MSG

CHAPTER 9

GOD WILL HELP ME

I walked into the grade school gym and saw the evil contraption. It was a thick heavy rope attached to the ceiling and hanging to the ground. Underneath was a cushioned mat. I knew what it meant, and I didn't like it. It meant utter humiliation for me. We were supposed to be able to climb at least partway up the rope. The first time we had to do it was when I was in third grade. I couldn't even get a foot up the rope.

After being laughed off the gym floor for failing, I took the option of walking the extra mile in fourth grade. This was fifth grade and the Presidential Fitness Challenge had come into being and was a requirement for every student. Mr. Benson,[1] the gym teacher, was a tall, large man wearing shorts. He said everyone had to try the climb at least twice if they didn't get up at least three feet the first time. If I couldn't do it one time, what would change by trying it a second time? I sighed heavily just thinking about it.

When my turn came, I hoped Mr. Benson would just call it quits but he didn't. He explained how to put my leg around the rope and how to pull myself up with my arms while pushing with my legs. Instead of climbing, though, I got my legs all tangled up in the rope and fell on the mat. It seemed everyone in the gym did a collective snicker. I heaved a big sigh and told the gym teacher I wasn't feeling well.

CLIMB THE ROPE OR ELSE

He said, "Ok but if you leave now, I will have to give you an F in gym class. If you try one more time, I'll give you an M for passing."

I looked around the room. Some were watching me, but not too many. I wanted to scream at Mr. Benson and run out of the room. Instead, I thought of the F on my report card and decided if they laughed at me once they could laugh again.

This time, Mr. Benson had a little more compassion and helped by supporting my feet with his foot, so I climbed the required height, got scared, let go and fell on the mat. He nodded as I asked permission to go to the restroom.

I truly hated exercise. There was nothing I liked about it.

I truly hated exercise. There was nothing I liked about it. Sure, I'd climbed a few feet, but Mr. Benson had helped me. The only other person he helped was short and fat Percy.[2] Mr. Benson hadn't even been able to help Percy get up a foot. There was no hope for Percy. I wasn't as bad as Percy, but that wasn't saying much.

When I came back to the gym, I had to do the pull-ups. I did one. Chin-ups, again I did one. I did 10 sit-ups. Then, I started walking around the gym to get in my mile. I knew I wouldn't make it the entire way. There wasn't time. Likely no one was watching me, but still, I hated exercise.

BIKE DISASTER

Maybe if they had a class where we rode bikes, I would like gym class. Bike riding was the one thing I enjoyed doing outside. Part of it was the freedom I felt whizzing down the road in front of our house. I'd join the kids in the neighborhood riding up and down our street.

Where we lived there were four small houses in a row with a church and its parking lot across the street. Beyond our four houses were about three blocks of open fields on either side of the road. The road sloped uphill at that point. We'd ride up to the top of the hill and then come down the road as fast as we could.

One summer afternoon, I was riding my bike feeling the freedom which only comes when the wind is in my hair and I'm speeding down the hill. I decided if I rode without my hands on the handlebars, I'd feel even freer. It was truly divine until I hit loose gravel from the parking lot at the bottom of the hill. In a split second, I got thrown off the bike. My head hit the pavement with such force Mom said she heard it inside the house. This was before safety helmets were a thing.

She came running outside and determined I needed stitches. Even though Mom had emotional issues, during emergencies she was calm, cool, collected and knew exactly what to do. She grabbed me and took me to the emergency room.

Later Dad teased me saying I had rocks in my head. The doctor did take out a rock which had been embedded in my forehead and did a few stitches. It wasn't as horrible as some of my own children's accidents, but it is one I remember.

Up until that point, I had loved riding bikes. I was about 14 when the accident happened and after then I rarely rode my bike. If I did, I held on tightly. It just never had the appeal it once had. I hadn't seen bike riding as exercise, it was just fun, until the bike disaster. Bike riding never again held the appeal it once had for me. It moved over to the category of an exercise I hated.

ICE-SKATING UPHEAVAL

I wasn't very good at roller skating, but I liked it, so when our church youth group decided to go to the ice-skating rink in a neighboring town, I was all for it. I'd never been ice skating before, but it couldn't be much more difficult than roller skating, right? Plus, our youth director said it was great fun, even better than roller skating.

We took a bus to the rink. At 13, I was one of the youngest going. I had no clue how to put on and lace up my skates. One of the sponsors gave me quick instructions and then headed out to the ice. I was left to lace up my skates and then get out to the rink. I watched others for a while before I attempted to stand on the slender blade, thankful I was holding on to the side.

As I was trying to pull myself along, one of the older guys asked if I wanted to skate with him. I told him I didn't know how.

"It's not hard," he said. "Just hold my hand. I'll help you."

I knew he was just trying to be nice. His girlfriend was a friend of mine. I decided to trust him. I skated with him about halfway around the rink. As long as I was holding on to him, I was fine. Then he just dropped my hand and skated off. It was his way of throwing me out into the water and letting me swim on my own, but I was too far away from the side of the rink and people were going way too fast around me. My one goal was to get to the side where I could hold on to a rail.

Then a speed skater whizzed past me and slightly touched me as he went around. I know he didn't do it to intentionally make me fall. He was basically letting me know he was there. One minute I was standing in the middle of the rink and the next I with my left foot underneath me.

After they figured out that I was indeed hurt and couldn't get up, a couple of guys helped me to the bench to take off my skates. My foot was swelling fast and hurt badly.

Everyone else ignored me and was having fun. Somehow it made sense the one time I went ice skating I would get hurt. When I finally got home, Dad wrapped my ankle with an ace bandage. We went to the doctor the next day and found I had a badly sprained ankle. He sent me home with crutches and told me to stay off of my foot for three weeks. Every time I took a step, it hurt and I was reminded of how much I hated exercise of any type.

HIGH SCHOOL GYM CLASS

In high school, we had some choices for gym class. One of those was swimming. I wished I could take swimming every semester, but I couldn't. I had to take the regular exercise class during the opposite semester.

It was hard enough walking around and around the grade school gym endless numbers of times to total up to a mile, but it was much worse walking the high school track. All the way around was a mile. If I was only halfway around and it was five minutes until the bell rang, I had to run. I don't like to run. When I run, I usually fall and hurt myself. We had about half an hour to walk the mile. Some even ran two miles during the same time. I was doing good if I made it a mile.

Swimming, though, was different. It was the one time I enjoyed going to gym class. It never felt like exercise. Although I wasn't a fast swimmer, I liked the sidestroke and backstroke. I loved being in the water. It felt peaceful. It was one exercise I enjoyed.

As an adult, any time anyone mentioned exercise I equated it with torture. I was glad I was done with physical education classes. I sincerely hoped those days were behind me. I didn't even like going shopping because I had to walk, and walking felt like exercise which was torture. Whenever I tried to lose weight and people would tell me I needed to exercise, I once again felt like I wanted to run and hide.

Any time anyone mentioned exercise I equated it with torture.

To be honest, I knew I had missed a lot of things when my children were growing up because I hadn't joined them and their dad on bike rides and hiking trips. Even when we'd go on vacation, they would go explore and I would sit in the car and read. I told them I preferred to read, but I just didn't want to walk. I knew exercise would be good for weight loss, but my experience taught me it was something I should avoid.

When I started on my lifestyle change journey, it was God who mentioned that nasty word to me again—exercise. One of the first concepts I learned was that instead of going on another diet to lose weight, I needed to learn how to change my habits. I needed to choose one bad habit to stop and a good habit to start. I just didn't realize the good habit would be exercise.

Instead of going on another diet, I needed to learn how to change my habits.

For habit change to work, I had to put firm boundaries around this bad habit. It wasn't something I was stopping temporarily until I got the weight off. It was a habit I wanted to discard completely. Stopping the bad habit would leave a void, so this meant I needed to start a good habit in its place. I would use all the energy I had been putting towards the thing I've just stopped to fuel this new and better habit which would help get me where I wanted to go.

I wanted to stop all sugar, but I knew this was not a doable stop for me. My stop had to be simpler so I would have success. I chose to stop eating candy. I knew what it was. I couldn't fool myself into saying I could eat it. Knowing it was childish would make it an easier thing for me to eliminate for the rest of my life.

The start was more challenging. This is when God dropped the bombshell and told me to start exercising. I argued with Him. I told Him I hated exercise. I told Him I got hurt exercising so how could it be good for me?

"Have you ever gotten hurt exercising in the water?" He asked. We had a family membership to our community recreation center which had a pool. I would go every once in a while to the water aerobics class. I hadn't been a regular, but I'd never gotten hurt in the water. The water supported my body. The more I thought about it, the more I knew the water was the best way for me to exercise.

I thought God would want me to take a Zumba, yoga or weight-lifting class, but He knows me. He knows what is best for me, what would work for me and what would help me the most on my journey. This was many years ago and I've been exercising in our community pool regularly ever since. It was the first good habit I started, and I still do it today, more than ten years later.

STRONGHOLD REVEALED

I didn't understand I had a stronghold where exercise was concerned. I thought I was just clumsy, accident-prone and no good at sports, but God helped me see moving is an integral part of working on my physical body, which is the very home of the Holy Spirit.

God helped me understand that my physical body is of importance to Him. It's where He lives and He doesn't want it filled with junk food wrappers. He wants to live in a fit and healthy body so together we can reach others with the message of His love.

Although in the beginning I began going to the pool for exercise, God has shown me my pool time does a lot more for me than exercise. I work from home and am in front of the computer a lot. My pool time helps me move, but it also gets me out of the house. I have to interact with real people even if it's just acknowledging they are there.

It also revives and refreshes me in a way I never dreamed possible. I love to go in the mornings before they begin playing music. It's just me and God jogging in the water. It's a time I look forward to. God knows He has my undivided attention when I'm there.

I started going three days a week for 30 minutes. As I added additional sugary things I wanted to stop, I added additional days and more time to exercise. These days I go five days a week. It's become a habit I don't want to miss.

I no longer hate exercise. I dearly love it. God addressed this lie I believed and turned it around simply by showing me the exercise which fits my lifestyle and helps me the most. I even do some recumbent bike riding and weightlifting from time to time.

Exercise has been an integral piece in my weight loss transformation. I had to get over my hatred and fear of it. God helped me change simply by sharing the truth with me that I've never been hurt while swimming. Working out in the water was an exercise I could do even when I was super morbidly obese. I am lighter in the water so, I am not taxing my joints as much.

HOW GOD HELPS ME

There are days when I don't want to go exercise because I don't feel like it, I have too much to do, the weather is bad or any number of reasons. On those days, I am reminded of what God said to me about my journey.

"Since we are surrounded by so great a cloud of witnesses, let us lay aside every weight, and the sin which so easily ensnares us, and let us run with endurance the race that is set before us, looking unto Jesus, the author and finisher of our faith, who for the joy that was set before Him endured the cross, despising the shame, and has sat down at the right hand of the throne of God."[3]

This is great encouragement for me because I want to lay aside every weight which holds me back. When I have committed to God to do something, I should not allow anything to keep me from it. It would be disobedience to God to do so. Disobedience is sin. Sin ensnares me and makes me falter on the race God has set before me.

This race a journey with Jesus as our guide. He's the one who started us on this path and the one who will be there at the end. Sometimes life gets hard. It even got hard for Jesus, but I love what these verses tell us. He didn't look at the pain

When it gets hard, we know He is with us helping us all the way.

or the shame of what was happening in the moment. He was always looking at the joy He knew awaited when He saw His Father once again. He endured everything He went through, even the horrible pain on the cross because He knew it was His purpose.

When it gets hard, we know He is with us helping us all the way. We need to remember this prescription to renew our spiritual vitality. "Be made strong even in your weakness by lifting up your tired hands in prayer and worship. And strengthen your weak knees, for as you keep walking forward on God's paths all your stumbling ways will be divinely healed!"[4]

God really has changed my desires. My exercise time is on my calendar. I work everything around it. The other day, Roy and I were having some car issues. He had an appointment out of town, and we were down to one car. I told him I would skip exercise.

He said, "I know how much you love to exercise. I don't want you to have to skip it. I'll take my motorcycle." He said this even though the forecast had a possibility of rain. It showed me God has helped me change completely in this area. Even Roy recognizes the change.

God knows us so much better than we know ourselves.

God helped me in an area I didn't even know I needed help. He's good at that. He knows us so much better than we know ourselves. "This plan of Mine is not what you would work out, neither are My thoughts the same as yours! For just as the heavens are higher than the earth, so are My ways higher than yours, and My thoughts than yours."[5]

I'm so glad I have a God who shares His thoughts and plans with me. His wisdom is what guides me on my journey. Thank You, God, for helping me navigate my life journey towards better health.

ENDNOTES

1. Not his real name.
2. Not his real name.
3. Hebrews 12:1-2 NKJV
4. Hebrews 12:12-13 TPT
5. Isaiah 55:8-9 TLB

"This plan of Mine is not what you would work out, neither are My thoughts the same as yours! For just as the heavens are higher than the earth, so are My ways higher than yours, and My thoughts than yours."

ISAIAH 55:8-9 TLB

CHAPTER 10

GOD ANSWERS
MY PRAYERS

Watching the Oral Roberts Show on television became a highlight of the week. I sat as close to the screen as possible, primarily because I didn't want to miss the time when he turned to the TV screen and spoke directly to me.

"Those of you watching by television can receive your miracle today," he said. "Just lay your hands on the TV screen while I pray." Then he'd pray for my personal miracle. I believed God could hear him. Every week I saw people walk across the stage and receive healing, shouting praises to God.

Growing up, I had one primary prayer request: Mom's healing. As early as I can remember this request topped every prayer list I ever made, the subject of every spoken and unspoken prayer request in church and Sunday School, the thing Grandma and I prayed for each time I spent the weekend with her and what Dad prayed for every night. With this much prayer going up on her behalf, I knew one day God might just get fed up with hearing her name and answer our prayers, so we'd all move on to something else.

139

Navigating Mom's moods was like walking through a forest of needles. I never knew when I'd step on something which would hurt me or her. I didn't understand why she was the way she was.

Dad said doctors were trying to help Mom, but only God could heal her. He told me often I needed to pray for her. I remember one time Dad left my brother and me with our grandparents for several weeks in the summer. Mom was going into the mental hospital. Dad and my grandparents were extremely upset about what was happening.

I think we need to pray because when we don't know what to do we should always pray.

Dad dropped us off and left. I remember sitting around the kitchen table with Grandma and Papaw. Grandma asked me about Mom, and I told her she was sick. Then, I started crying. Grandma reached for my hand and I saw she was crying too.

Papaw said, "I think we need to pray because when we don't know what to do, we should always pray." He led us in a long prayer. By the end, he was crying too. It's the first time I had ever seen Papaw cry. I realized then how sad they must have felt as her parents.

I kept praying for her, but it seemed her behaviors got worse instead of better. About the time I was 12, Mom had gotten so bad she didn't want to go to church and she didn't want Dad to leave her on Sunday morning. Dad sent my brother, sister and I across the street to a different church where he knew the pastor. Any time prayer requests were taken, I asked for prayer for Mom. It was the only thing I ever asked for. Those in my church felt sorry for me because they knew she didn't come to church and she was sick.

PRAYER WARRIOR

They probably knew what her issue was better than I did. They continued to pray. Betty was a prayer warrior who went to my church and also lived in our neighborhood. She often would tell me she was praying for Mom. It was a source of comfort for me to know she was praying not just at church but other times as well.

All of my extended family and any friends we had were all praying for her too. Because like Dad said, "God is the only one who can heal her." I just wished He'd hurry up and do it. I mean if He could heal her, why was it taking so long? Was her case so hard even God couldn't heal her?

This went on until the summer before I was ready to leave for college. I wanted to go away for college even though we had great universities in my hometown. I knew I could not live at home and get any studying done. I needed to leave.

At the same time, I was concerned about my siblings' safety. I had accidentally read a letter Mom had written to Oral Roberts asking for prayer. The things she said she had recently contemplated doing greatly concerned me because they didn't just involve her. They also involved my brother and sister. What she wrote might just have been a cry for help, but still, it jolted me into realizing how far she had fallen into the abyss which had become her life.

I talked to Dad about it and he said, "Your job is to go to college. My job is to look after your mother, brother and sister." He reassured me things would be fine and he'd make sure

Randy and Renee were safe. I breathed a sigh of relief. I trusted he would protect them. I decided I could go to college as long as I stayed in touch with him to get updates.

Towards the end of the summer, I saw Betty in the hall of the newspaper office where we both worked.

"Teresa, when are you leaving for school?" she said smiling and hugging me.

I leaned into her but didn't return the hug or answer her question. I wasn't in a good mood.

She added as she turned to walk away, "I just want you to know I'm praying for your Momma."

Mom still found her way to the top of my prayer list.

I furrowed my brow and grabbed her arm. Even the lines of wisdom etched in her face and her smiling eyes couldn't deter me from what I was about to say to her. "Don't pray for Mom anymore. God isn't going to answer. I've prayed for her for 18 years and I've had no indication He has heard me once. There's no reason to pray. Don't waste your breath."

Fury rising inside, I stalked out the door like the stubborn, angry teenager I was. Even as I did that, I was sure Betty added me to her prayer list.

Though I vowed not to pray for Mom, when I got to college she still found her way to the top of my prayer list. On my frequent calls home, I talked with Dad who gave me most of the news, but he always sounded so tired. Mom's mood swings varied widely so she never wanted to talk.

The astounding call came early in November from Mom. "Teresa are you sitting down?" she said in a calm voice.

"What's up, Mom?"

"Jesus healed me."

"What?"

"Jesus healed me." I didn't know what to say. Over the next few minutes, she and Dad told me an incredible story.

Mom had gotten so bad she would not go out of the house. She wouldn't go to church, the store, even to a friend's house. Yvonne, a woman from a church in another city where Mom and Dad attended more than 15 years before, called Mom out of the blue.

"There is a Full Gospel Businessmen's Fellowship Meeting in your town tonight," she said. "I'll be at your house by 6:30 p.m. to pick you up."

Miraculously Mom agreed to go even though it had been months since she had been anywhere. At the meeting, the evangelist spoke about emotional illness. After the message, he said, "There are three people here tonight whom God is going to touch. I want you to stand."

HANGING ON TO JESUS

Mom and two other people stood. The preacher spoke to each one individually. To Mom, he said, "God touched you tonight and started your healing process. For it to continue, you must fit your life into God's word rather than fitting God's word into your life.

"Read God's word for what it really says and do that. Don't try to find an excuse or to take any verse out of context to do what you want to do. God sent His word. It has healing power and life. Read it under the inspiration and guidance of the Holy

Spirit. Ask God to open your heart to really understanding what it says."

I knew Mom tended to try to use the Bible to her advantage and twisting the words around to permit herself to do certain things. So, I asked, "Mom, so what are you going to do?"

She said, "I'm going to hang on to Jesus as tight as I can."

At Thanksgiving she was a different person. She started a journey that continued until the day she died. Though she had some difficulties, each day got better.

The next time I saw Betty, I threw my arms around her and hugged her for a long time. I apologized for my insolent attitude and thanked her for never giving up praying for Mom.

"I serve a God who always answers prayer," she said. "Our job is to keep praying and have just a little more faith than we did before."

WALKING IT OUT

I was privileged to watch Mom begin her transformation. I watched her hang on tight to Jesus. I watched her walk out her healing. The preacher was right. It wasn't instantaneous, but I heard from Dad how she started having Bible study and prayer with him every morning.

She went back to church with him, going to every service he did. She began taking up new hobbies, volunteering and helping several of her friends who also had mental health issues. She cared for several babies and toddlers, usually no more than one or two at a time. She loved working with kids.

I watched her work out her own salvation with fear and trembling. Scripture says it this way. "Now you must continue to make this new life fully manifested as you live in the holy awe of God—which brings you trembling into His presence. God will continually revitalize you, implanting within you the passion to do what pleases Him."[1]

She got so much better that when Dad got ordained, she was right there with him. When he started doing interim pastor work or even guest preaching, she was with him all the way. Eventually, he pastored a small church. She saw the need for something for the kids, so she developed and led a children's church program.

TRUSTING MOM

Somewhere in there, my siblings and I all got married. She would often tell me and my sister that she and Dad were praying for grandchildren. Her prayers were answered when my son was born and less than a year later, my sister's first daughter was born.

Mom agreed to babysit my newborn son and I was elated he would be staying with someone who loved him. I had no reservations. She was also babysitting my cousin's daughter. When I was growing up if you had told me I would trust Mom to take care of one of my children I would have said you were crazy. It's just amazing what miracles God can do in a person's life.

Unfortunately, Mom contracted colon cancer when Andrew was four. She had to stop babysitting to manage the awful disease. I became pregnant with my daughter soon after that. Jenny was only two when Mom died in 1992.

During all of this time, I had been steadily gaining weight. Eventually, I got to the point where I hit rock bottom. I needed to figure out how to overcome my addiction to sugar but giving up sugar still felt like an impossible task.

FOLLOWING MOM'S EXAMPLE

The night this all hit me, I began thinking about Mom. She had faced an impossible circumstance as well. Overcoming a mental and emotional illness was impossible without God's help.

Then I remembered what she told me. She said, "I'm going to hang on to Jesus as tight as I can." I watched her do that. I figured if she could walk out her journey with God's help, I could, too. So that's what I did.

There's more to it but in reality, holding tight to Jesus is the only thing to get us through something which has become a stronghold in our lives. Emotional illness was a stronghold in Mom's life. The preacher also told her not to stop her medications, but to find a psychiatrist who would work with her to reduce her medicines and help her understand and deal with her emotions.

> I'm going to hang on to Jesus as tight as I can.

In the past, the doctors and hospitals she had gone to were simply trying to medicate her to fix her issue. Mom needed a different strategy. She needed Someone more powerful than her to be her guide. Like Mom, I had tried every diet imaginable to fix me. I didn't need a diet or medication to fix me. I needed to allow God to lead me every step of the way.

I saw how much like Mom I had been. I wanted to do things my way. I wanted to try to think, worry and plan my way to lose weight and still eat what I wanted. Mom had tried to think, worry and plan her way to avoiding life, which is what she thought she wanted.

Mom didn't want to avoid life. She just couldn't figure out how to navigate her way back into life. In the same way, I didn't want to eat everything in sight, I just couldn't figure out how to control my emotions without trying to eat them away.

LETTING GO OF LIES

I finally saw what I needed to do. I had to let go of the lies I believed about God. One of the big ones was God wouldn't answer my prayers. God had dispelled this lie, though, hadn't He? He had answered the prayer for Mom, but had He answered my prayer? Had He healed me of my obesity?

I heard God say to me, "I can't heal you of obesity because you are holding tightly to what you want. I have given you freedom and you have chosen to spend it on your own pleasures. You have chosen to eat what you want when you want. It has always been your choice and, My Daughter. It still is."

I was focused on my selfish desires[2] of eating whatever I wanted whenever I wanted. The truth was, God had answered my prayer way back in 1977 when He told me exactly what I should eat and not eat. If I had done what He told me to do back then, I wouldn't be in the predicament I was in.

WALKING OUT MY JOURNEY

Sugar had become my drug of choice, but the preacher told Mom to not get off of her medicines all at once but to work with someone to help her titrate off the wrong medications and get on the right ones. I had to do the same. I wanted to give up all sugar, but I knew if I did that, I'd just go back to eating it again. I'd fall off the wagon and beat myself up and placate those emotions by overeating. I was done with that. I needed a different way.

In Russ I found a mentor to help me learn how to change my habits and start on the road to recovery. Now I live a fasted lifestyle. I don't eat foods that contain processed sugar or flour. Every time I give up those kinds of foods, I do it as unto the Lord. I see it as my sacrifice of praise. It took me time to get to this place, but the beautiful benefit of knowing every day I am walking hand-in-hand with Jesus outweighs any of the difficulties, trials and heartaches I've had getting here.

> The beautiful benefit of knowing every day that I am walking hand-in-hand with Jesus outweighs any of the difficulties I've had getting here.

To live any other way would mean I have willfully chosen to put myself back in bondage to sugar and food addiction. "Let me be clear, the Anointed One has set us free—not partially, but completely and wonderfully free! We must always cherish this truth and stubbornly refuse to go back into the bondage of our past."[3]

I used to stubbornly refuse to give up the foods I loved. The desire for those foods became a stronghold that held me in bondage. These days I am stubborn about approaching anything which even looks or smells like it is going to put me back in bondage.

The best thing is now I am completely free to follow wherever Jesus leads me. The devil may come knocking at my door. He may try to capture me in his sly schemes, but nothing tastes as good as the freedom Christ brings feels. Nothing! "I will walk with You in complete freedom, for I seek to follow Your every command."[4]

CHOOSING CHANGE

To say God doesn't answer our prayers may seem like truth because He rarely answers them in the way we want Him to. He won't force change on us. He asks us to choose change. He will lead us to complete freedom, but we have to listen to His direction and follow His guidance. Otherwise, we will find ourselves in bondage to things we wish we could break free from. These things seep in slowly and before we know it, we have allowed a stronghold to take over.

James tells us how to let God break any stronghold. "So let God work His will in you. Yell a loud no to the devil and watch him scamper. Say a quiet yes to God and He'll be there in no time. Quit dabbling in sin. Purify your inner life. Quit playing the field. Hit bottom and cry your eyes out. The fun and games are over. Get serious, really serious. Get down on your knees before the Master; it's the only way you'll get on your feet."[5]

We don't have to worry about what we've done in the past because God will show us how to break our strongholds. All we have to do is stop listening to the evil one's lies and surrender completely to God.

God answered my prayers for Mom, and He answered my prayers regarding my own journey. Neither answer came in the timeframe or the way I had envisioned, but He did answer.

I shouldn't have been surprised about either answer. John tells us, "We are confident that He hears us whenever we ask for anything that pleases Him. And since we know He hears us when we make our requests, we also know that He will give us what we ask for."[6]

God hears us and He answers us when we ask anything which pleases Him. Another translation says, "We can also have great boldness before Him, for if we present any request agreeable to His will, He will hear us."[7] Still, another adds, "If we ask anything that is consistent with His plan and purpose, He hears us."[8]

God answers our prayers for how we can walk in total health.

What is in His will? I can say without a doubt one thing that is in His will is for His children to follow health—physically, mentally, emotionally and spiritually. He answers our prayers for how we can walk total health.

It may not be the miraculous, instant deliverance we want. Sometimes we won't even recognize He has answered our prayers until later, but He does hear, and He does answer. I know because I have experienced it.

The lesson I learned is to keep praying and be ready for His answer, no matter what it is. He will answer. We just have to recognize His voice, listen and follow where He leads. Following is always where we tend to miss the mark, but He will keep working with us.

Just when I thought for sure He had stopped trying to help me on my weight loss journey, He answered me. Thank God, I finally listened and followed. He is my biggest advocate and very best counselor.

ENDNOTES

1. Phil 2:12-13 TPT
2. Romans 13:14 TPT
3. Galatians 5:1 TPT
4. Psalm 119:45 TPT
5. James 4:7-10 MSG
6. 1 John 5:14-15 NLT
7. 1 John 5:14 TPT
8. 1 John 5:14 AMP

"I will walk with You in complete freedom, for I seek to follow Your every command."

PSALM 119:45 TPT

CHAPTER 11

HOLY SPIRIT IS MY COMFORTER

After working with God to tear down many of the mental strongholds which led me to become a sugar addict, surrendering my addiction to God and following what He showed me to do, I began losing weight. I was finally headed in the right direction and the weight was staying off. I had processed and dealt with many lies that had held me back for years. I felt good about myself for the first time in a very long time.

When I'd start to lose weight previously, I was waiting for everything to fall apart. This feeling was now gone, and I was thanking God. No longer were sugar, desserts and comfort foods ruling my life. It was such a welcome relief.

Then, I hit a brick wall. It came out of nowhere. I tried everything to fix it, but nothing was working.

I was at the 200-pound mark and I so wanted to go into one-derland. I had been steadily losing weight, but when I would see 199 on the scale, I could feel myself panic. Instead of being happy, I was afraid something was wrong.

I was exercising five days a week for an hour. I was eating all the right things and none of the wrong things, but the scale just wouldn't move any lower. The next day I'd be back to 200 pounds and for some reason, I would feel myself internally breathe a sigh of relief. It was an internal struggle, but I couldn't figure out the source.

I knew there was a lie somewhere which was keeping me stuck, but I had no idea what it was or even where to look. I kept trying to figure out what I was doing wrong. Maybe my body just needs to rest from losing weight? Maybe I am at a plateau? Maybe I'm eating too little and my body thinks it's in starvation mode? Maybe I'm eating too much and I need to cut back? Maybe I need to add more vegetables or protein? Addressing all of these still did nothing to change my weight.

STRANGE QUESTION

I was attending my weekly accountability meeting with others who were on weight loss journeys. It was facilitated by Russ. For the last several weeks I hadn't mentioned my issue. I just hadn't reported any weight loss. This week I decided to come clean and report what was going on.

The members all gave me input about what to try. These were things I had already tried. I didn't want to leave the meeting without some direction, but I resigned myself to think this might just be where my body wanted to stay. I wasn't happy with the idea, but I wasn't sure what else to do.

Russ had been sitting back listening to everything being said. Then, he asked me a question that seemed totally unrelated to what I had just shared. "Where did you learn your relationship with food?" His question invaded my mind. I had been in defense mode assuring everyone I had done everything under the sun to break this plateau. Now he was requiring me to dig deep.

I didn't have to stop and think, "Do I have a relationship with food?" We are not supposed to have a relationship with food. We have relationships with people, but not with food. Food, even fresh food, isn't alive. Its job is to give us fuel for our bodies. We don't have a relationship with the gas in our cars. We shouldn't have a relationship with food, but none of those thoughts went through my mind at the time.

> I didn't have to stop and think, "Do I have a relationship with food?"

I immediately knew I had a relationship with food, and I knew I learned it from Grandma who fed me with every kind of food I wanted including every type of dessert. There were seconds or thirds and we could have snacks at any time.

COMFORT FOOD

I preferred Grandma's more lavish food style to Mom's three balanced meals a day. Supper at our house was very regimented. If Mom cooked, she would prepare just enough for one portion for each of us. Dessert would usually be a can of fruit cocktail divided between us.

Most of the time the meat would be fish sticks, hamburgers or hot dogs. Every once in a while, we would have pork chops or roast, but only if Papaw had given us the meat. Liver, though, was the bane of my existence. She insisted on serving liver once a week. We didn't have to eat it, but we wouldn't get our fruit if we didn't. I couldn't stand to even smell it.

We could not sneak snacks at home. Still, I risked getting a spanking to steal caramels from the bag Mom kept on the top shelf in the kitchen. It was totally different at Grandma's house. What kid wouldn't want to be able to eat as much dessert as they wanted any time they wanted?

Grandma's way of handling food felt like comfort and love. When I was away from her and felt overwhelmed, sad, angry, lonely, fearful, worried, stressed or just plain old frustrated, I would make something she would have made and eat as much as I wanted. It would comfort me for a while until the sugar-high wore off. Then I needed more to get the same feeling.

To not ever again eat or cook those foods felt like I would be dishonoring Grandma.

In reality, this way of coping wasn't comforting at all. It was very discomforting. It had caused me to gain weight and then struggle through learning how to lose that weight. To not ever again eat or cook those foods felt like I would be dishonoring Grandma. It took me a while to process what was happening in my head and heart.

I knew Grandma didn't aim to hurt me. She fed me out of love, but those foods were harming me. This saddened me because I knew it would also make Grandma sad if she were still alive.

While the adult me knew I couldn't eat all of those foods in the quantities I had consumed in the past and be healthy, the emotional part of me was still stuck back baking cookies with

Grandma. I had equated those foods with love and comfort. They fed my emotions more than my body.

All of a sudden God revealed the truth to me. I had allowed Grandma's way of cooking to become a stronghold. It was robed in what I thought was comfort, but it was still a stronghold. Grandma's comfort food had become my legacy. This had become more deeply embedded in me after both she and Mom died within six months of each other. I felt the responsibility to pass on what Grandma taught me.

> Grandma and the comfort foods she cooked had become enmeshed in my heart. Could I separate them?

The main things she had left me were her recipes. Those recipes carried reminders of great family dinners and celebrations. I put together *Grandma's Kitchen Cookbook* so my family members could all have copies of recipes from all the great cooks in our family, but the legacy I wanted to share the most was Grandma's.

My fondest childhood memories all center around food and Grandma. They were inseparable in my mind. I thought if I gave up throwing the grand food celebrations Grandma was famous for, I would be dishonoring her legacy. I had equated Grandma's legacy with the comfort foods she cooked. They had become enmeshed in my heart. Could I separate them? Could I still hold a place in my heart for Grandma if I turned my back on what she cooked and served?

By this time, I wasn't eating the type of things I remember Grandma making, but I couldn't imagine never again cooking her hot rolls, chocolate pie, brownies, oatmeal cake or myriads of other special dishes for others.

GRANDMA'S LOVE

After sharing what I had discovered, Russ asked, "What would your grandmother say to you if she knew certain foods were causing you to ruin your health?"

I knew she would tell me to give them up. I remember her saying to me, "Honey, you would be so pretty and feel so much better if you would lose some weight." Five minutes later, she would say, "I baked a batch of oatmeal cookies. Eat as many as you want." The second message always drowned out the first.

Many people show their love for their families through the food they cook. Grandma was no exception. It was her way of showing love, but it wasn't the only way. I remember her reading my favorite book, *Henny Penny*, over and over again. I loved the rhythm of the words.

Any time I spent with Grandma was a time I treasured.

At the end of the day, we'd sit outside under the oak tree with Papaw and watch the traffic pass by. Many times, friends would pull in the drive and come sit with us for a while to pass the time. Grandma and I would be sitting as close together as possible. I might be helping her snap beans or shell peas. Any time I spent with Grandma was a time I treasured.

My favorite time with her, though, was when we'd go to sleep at the end of the day. She would make me a pallet down beside her bed. She'd reach her hand down to hold mine until I fell asleep. I loved those times because I also got to hear her and Papaw pray together before going to sleep. It made me feel wrapped in love since they always prayed for me and every member of the family. I knew they did that every night. It was a comfort better than any food could bring.

God used those moments after Russ asked me what Grandma would think of my weight loss to begin destroying the mental stronghold which drove me to believe if I lost any more weight, I would be dishonoring Grandma.

Grandma was a large woman. I don't know what she weighed, but I know she weighed at least 200 pounds. She had soft mushy parts perfect for grandkids to crawl up in her lap, fall into her and feel loved. My emotions were telling me if I became smaller than Grandma had been and wasn't fixing the foods she fixed, I was rejecting her.

> My emotions were telling me if I became smaller than Grandma had been and wasn't fixing the foods she fixed, I was rejecting her.

Finally, I saw the truth I'd been missing all of my life. Mom, the one whose way of feeding us felt cold and unemotional, was trying to show us the right way to eat. She was showing us love in an entirely different way. She had studied home economics in high school and had learned how to serve balanced meals. She went against her mother's way of cooking and did not cook too much food.

Grandma was cooking the way her mother had cooked and probably her mother before her. Mom realized she wasn't cooking for a farm family. Even though Dad worked hard, he wasn't working 12 to 16 hours a day from sunup to sundown in the fields.

Mom was trying to show us a better way. She was showing us her version of love by teaching us to eat healthily. When she made liver and onions and told us we had to eat it before we could have our fruit for dessert, she was trying to help us. Liver has iron in it. Even today I'm low on iron and take iron supplements.

As a kid, I thought she was just being mean. Grandma's way of letting me eat as many cookies as I wanted anytime I wanted felt like an extravagant show of love, but Mom was loving me in her way. I just didn't get it until it was almost too late

Destroying this stronghold came after breaking through many other strongholds. It was one of the last ones I encountered, but it was huge because it carried so much emotion with it.

When strongholds are wrapped in those we love, it is hard to separate the lie from the one we love.

When I saw the truth of what I had been believing, I realized how the enemy can use even the most loving memories to set up lies which become some of the fiercest strongholds.

When they are wrapped in those we love and cherish, it is hard to separate the lie from the one we love. It is in separating the lies from the person that the stronghold crumbles.

It wasn't an automatic breaking, like a lightning bolt breaking a tree in half. It was more like watching someone saw limbs off the tree one at a time from the top down until the stump is finally blasted out of the ground. I knew when the blast happened to me because it caused an emotional, tearful response. There were so many things in my past which had to be redefined; it felt like I was losing a part of me.

Seeing my past in an entirely new light, though, was like seeing a rainbow and sunset all at the same time. It was such a new experience. Now when I think about Grandma, I picture her as engulfing me in the kind of hug which only she could give. I feel love cascading from her every pore. She was the epitome of comfort to me and our entire family. She brought us all together. Family togetherness was her gift.

I also have a renewed respect for what Mom was trying to do for us. Because of her illness, it was hard for me to see her way of dealing with food was better, even more concerned and loving than Grandma's.

GENERATIONAL CURSES?

Many of us have this stronghold especially if we grew up with mothers or grandmothers who were great cooks. We can't give up the comfort foods loved ones cooked because we feel it is our legacy and maybe the only connection to our past.

In many ways, it may seem to dishonor those we loved to not cook family recipes anymore no matter how unhealthy they are. Giving this up is easy once we realize it's more important for us and our family to live and be healthy than continue a tradition that is killing us.

If we continue to cook and eat this way, we are perpetuating what many call a generational curse. What people are referring to when they use these words to define the problem with certain diseases like diabetes, high blood pressure, heart disease and obesity is a lifestyle of eating which has been passed down through the generations. We cook what Grandma cooked because it's what we remember and what we know. We continue to cook it because she did even though it is unhealthy for us and our families.

These days I no longer cook what I consider legacy recipes and have changed the way I do family dinners when we gather at my house. I don't make five different desserts. I have a fresh fruit salad, a lettuce salad, vegetables and meat. If others want other dishes, they bring them. We have enough to eat and there are always healthy options.

The legacy I want to leave is one of health and love.

This may seem like a logical solution and it is, but it took a long time for me to get there, especially coming from feeling love oozing out of every meal Grandma prepared. Our family still makes it a point to show we care for each other. When we get together, we do things like art projects, games of all types and fun activities. Food is no longer the focus. Breaking this stronghold wasn't hard when I finally came to my own truth. The legacy I want to leave is one of health and love.

WHAT IS COMFORT?

Comfort food isn't true comfort. True comfort only comes from the Holy Spirit. Jesus explained this to His disciples before He was crucified, "I will pray the Father, and He shall give you another Comforter, that He may abide with you forever; even the Spirit of truth; whom the world cannot receive, because it seeth Him not, neither knoweth Him: but ye know Him; for

He dwelleth with you, and shall be in you. I will not leave you comfortless: I will come to you."[1]

I love the way the King James Version uses the word Comforter to describe the Holy Spirit, who is the Spirit of Christ. We receive the Holy Spirit when we accept Christ. It's the Holy Spirit inside us who gives us true comfort. He can quiet our souls. He can ease our pain. He can whisper words of encouragement to us. He can lead us into everything God wants for us.

We have access to the supreme Comforter. Why do we need or want anything else?

We need comfort. We can't do without it, but it must be the comfort the Holy Spirit brings. Everything else is just placating our soulish and selfish desires. Jesus came to free us from ourselves. Sending the Holy Spirit to live inside us seals the deal. We have access to the supreme Comforter. Why do we need or want anything else?

The Psalmist declared, "When I screamed out, 'Lord, I'm doomed' Your fiery love was stirred, and You raced to my rescue. Whenever my busy thoughts were out of control, the soothing comfort of Your presence calmed me down and overwhelmed me with delight."[2] There is just nothing like God's presence to comfort us. It is better than the finest dessert Grandma ever made.

Real comfort is knowing God is on our side. He will never leave us. He is planning our future. He has everything all worked out. We don't have to stress or worry. We can leave it in His hands, and it will be all right. There is nothing more comforting to me than knowing this truth.

The barrier I felt at the 200-pound weight mark was an emotional one and it was real. Even my body didn't want to compete with Grandma. It was stubbornly holding on to the weight. Confronting the feeling of I am not honoring Grandma when I lose more than what she weighed, freed me to be the person God wants me to be. It broke the stronghold which said I have to serve Grandma's recipes for my family to be comforted.

> I am free to be the person God wants me to be.

Breaking this stronghold freed me to continue to lose weight and love being me. It freed me to embrace becoming healthy. It freed me to be able to cook things that won't contribute to others being unhealthy. It freed me to love my family in the right way and not by filling them full of foods that lead them toward an early grave.

It freed me to reprioritize my memories of Grandma to include the wonderful woman she was and not just the foods she cooked. It freed me to be me. It freed me to follow God in all things.

ENDNOTES

1. John 14:16-18 KJV
2. Psalm 94:18-19 TPT

CHAPTER 12

GOD KNOWS ME

Every year, Grandma would select a poem for me to memorize and recite during the Christmas program at Mt. Gilead Baptist Church. She loved having me perform and I loved learning and reciting the poems she picked for me. The year I was 12, Grandma decided since I did such a good job learning one poem a year, she would have me learn and recite two poems.

The small country church was jam-packed with people for the Christmas program. I'm not sure if it was because I'd never seen that many people there or because I was 12 and suddenly self-conscious, but I looked at the crowd and realized everyone was watching me. My mind went blank after five verses of the first six-verse poem. I couldn't remember the last verse. I stopped and tried not to look at the multitude of eyes staring back at me.

There were words in my head, but I knew they were from the other poem. I stood frozen center stage in my black and red plaid dress with black patent leather shoes and white socks.

Grandma was in the front row trying to tell me the next line, but she didn't have the poem with her, and I knew the words she was mouthing were not correct.

As a sea of faces stared back, I ran off the stage, down the center aisle, past all the people and out the back door to the safety of the huge oak tree. It's where I remember Grandma reading Vacation Bible School stories to me and several other kids. This day, though, was not a balmy, summer day. It was beyond freezing.

I didn't want her to see the tears frozen on my face.

Tears streamed down my cheeks. All I could remember was the shocked look on Grandma's face as I ran down the aisle past her. I stayed out there for a long time. I guess Grandma thought I was at the back of the church. She did not come to find me, and I was glad. I didn't want her to see the tears freezing on my face. It felt as if something special had been stolen from me. I didn't know exactly what it was, but I knew I couldn't stand to see those faces again.

There under the oak tree, I swore I would never speak in front of an audience again. I never wanted to feel that level of embarrassment and shame. For years I kept the oath. It wasn't hard. I would want to speak, and I'd be fine until I got on stage. Then I would begin shaking, perspiring and feeling like I would throw up.

I remember one time my former church was having an anniversary celebration. I was working for a denominational headquarters as a writer. The church asked me to talk about the work I was doing and the various jobs I'd had. I thought, sure why not?

I didn't think too much about it. I was planning on going anyway. I was a self-assured adult woman. I thought I could do it until I stepped up to the podium and was sure I was going to be sick. I looked out at the people, many of whom I'd known since childhood, and my mind went blank. I don't know what I said, but it wasn't what I had written on the paper in front of me because those words just blurred together.

Again, I vowed no matter how much logical sense it made for me to speak somewhere, I would remember this day and the day at Mt. Gilead Baptist Church. Clearly, I was not meant to speak. I didn't have a voice for speaking. I had one for writing, but not for speaking. Speaking definitely wasn't my forte. The evil one didn't have to do much to convince me. I could see it by my track record and the fear which rose in me every time I tried to speak.

THE FREEDOM EXPERIENCE

In 1994 I was part of a freedom seminar with Russ as the director. One exercise was to memorize and lip-sync a song in front of the group. We were to be "judged" by those in the seminar. They would stand when they experienced us being real. I had no idea this was part of the seminar when I signed up.

When I heard what I was going to have to do my fear of being in performance mode was heightened. Not only would I be in front of people and parading all of my fat, but I was going to be judged. I had gotten through some of the other harder parts and this was to be one of the final activities before graduating. I didn't want to be a quitter. Still the 12-year old girl inside me wanted to find that oak tree quickly.

My time came to perform. There was no backing out. I knew the song. I had to do this. The minute the first strains of "You Light Up My Life" started, I could feel myself shaking. At the end of the first verse and into the chorus, those in front of me were still sitting down and I began to shake even more realizing if they didn't stand, I'd have to go through this entire mortifying ritual again.

The chorus was simple. "You light up my life, you give me hope to carry on. You light up my days and fill my nights with song." As I sang the words, I started pointing to each person, looking them in the eyes. To my amazement as I did that, they began to stand one by one.

The trainers, though, still weren't standing. I had to get them all to stand to not have to do this again. Through the next verse and into the chorus I began pointing to each trainer and they began standing. At the final chorus, the group began pointing back at me.

I sang the rest of the song through a veil of tears not caring what was happening or who was standing or not standing. As I cried, I noticed I wasn't alone. Their tears were joining with mine. I looked up to see Russ standing on top of a table joining me as tears streamed down his face. Somehow, I knew being in front of people would never be a huge problem again.

TRANSFORMATIONAL LEADER

Fast forward a few more years and I was in Russ' in-depth seminar called Transformational Leader. Even though the other workshop helped dispel my fear of physically being in front of a crowd, it didn't do anything to remove the fear of having to speak in front of a group again. The lie of I don't have a voice was still there.

This workshop had about 20 people, all leaders or aspiring leaders. It was a four-month workshop. We'd meet for several days and then get assignments for the next time we met which would be in about three weeks. This time the next assignment was to develop a five to seven-minute talk on our life manifesto or mission.

The lie of I don't have a voice was still there.

This felt monumental. I thought about it, wrote about it and prayed about it for most of the next three weeks. My biggest fear was falling flat on my face in front of all the members. I was no longer afraid to stand up in front of everyone, but I also didn't want to be seen as a failure. I figured if I could write out my speech and read it, everything would be fine.

On the day we were to start giving our speeches, Russ called up the first person. He came prepared with his talk typed out. Then Russ walked up to him and asked for the paper. Russ said, "Speak from your heart. What is your life mission?"

I was mortified for the young man and for me. This meant I couldn't read what I had written. I had to speak without a net. I had to find my voice. Fear grabbed hold of me again reminding me of how I felt standing in front of Grandma's packed country church and messing up my lines. I didn't want to make a fool of myself once again.

Gently, the Holy Spirit reminded me of the other workshop where everyone stood for me. This experience had helped me understand even more deeply how much God shows His perfect love to me through others. I just wasn't sure how it would work this time. I wasn't lip-syncing a song. I was talking. What if nothing came out of my mouth? What if I truly had no voice?

Within the timespan we were supposed to spend together for the Transformational Leader workshop, we needed to get a good start towards building our life mission by working on one of our dreams. We also needed to have an idea of when the first phase of this could be completed.

My real dream was to write a book, but I had no idea what that book would be about.

During the very first meeting, three young men declared they were going to write books on specific topics. My real dream was to write a book, but I had no idea what that book would be about.

How could I develop such a dream without any idea of the subject of the book? I had no clear vision and no action steps. It wasn't something I could accomplish or even start in five months.

I still wanted to write, so I decided I'd change my specific dream I'd work on from writing a book to developing an online publication. I had a blog, but it was on a free site that didn't allow advertising. I knew if I did an online magazine, I'd eventually want to have a way to sell things on the website. This meant my first step would be to figure out where to transfer my blog and create an actual website. At least I had a step towards doing something.

Writing real stories about real people encountering a real God became my project. During my talk I discussed the importance of sharing people's stories of the overcoming power of God. I talked about how writing makes me come alive. It came straight from my heart without notes. There was no shaking or quivering. I got through it without being sick to my stomach. It seemed maybe I did have a tiny voice after all.

TRANSFORMATIVE PROCESS

I continued writing blogs and stories, but soon it was clear God had a different purpose for the website I set up during the workshop. By October of 2013, I had published my first book, *Sweet Grace.* I also changed the name of my website to my author name and began using it, along with my social media platforms to share about my book.

When I attended a reunion of the Transformation Leader participants in 2014, I was the only one who had written and published a book during the two years since we had met. I confessed I had been too intimidated by the others' specifics about books they were going to write to even mention it had been my dream since childhood to write a book.

Being a part of the group rekindled my pursuit of writing. This led me to publish my first book and begin the amazing journey I am on. It would have never happened had I not been challenged to decide to take one step towards something I wanted to pursue in my life. Russ asked all the right questions and got my brain motivated to take action again. He challenged the stronghold which screamed to me I don't have a voice and can't speak in public.

> Confronting this lie broke the stronghold.

Confronting this lie broke the stronghold. I didn't realize this phenomenal shift had happened. I was just happy I was able to talk in front of a group. It wasn't something I thought

I'd ever be doing. Public speaking still wasn't on my bucket list. God, though, had different plans. Doesn't He always?

TESTING MY VOICE

In August 2013, I was talking to Wendy about a release date and launch party for *Sweet Grace*. "You do know this means you need to speak at this event, right?" she asked.

I said, "Oh no, not me. I have several people who can speak. I'll just listen."

She said, "They are coming to hear your story. You can have a few others say some words, but you have to be the main speaker."

This was the first time I had even considered that writing a book might mean I'd have to start speaking. I was so focused on writing the book it had never crossed my mind. On the day of the book launch party, even though I had copious notes on my iPad, I spoke from my heart and loved every moment of it. The words flowed effortlessly.

Writing a book meant I had to speak about it.

I realized the stronghold which says I can't speak in public was broken. This only happened with God's help.

From birth, He knew me. He "watched me as I was being formed in utter seclusion, as I was woven together in the dark of the womb. You saw me before I was born. Every day of my life was recorded in Your book. Every moment was laid out before a single day had passed."[1]

172

He knew my purpose before I was even born and has been weaving together my storyline all this time. Even when I threw plot twists in there, He still knew what to do to get me to my destiny.

"We are convinced that every detail of our lives is continually woven together to fit into God's perfect plan of bringing good into our lives, for we are His lovers who have been called to fulfill His designed purpose."[2]

God knows me. He knew the day would come when my voice would be more than words on paper. I am more than mystified at how He got me to the place where I am no longer afraid to speak.

He knew one day my voice would be heard at workshops and seminars, in my coaching group and courses I have developed, but God wouldn't stop there. My voice would be heard on national and international Christian television stations, radio, Facebook lives, Instagram, Pinterest, YouTube and even my own podcast. He had a plan to make it all happen before I ever desired to utter a word.

> God knew one day my voice would be heard at workshops and seminars, in my coaching group and courses I have developed.

The Psalmist said, "You know what I am going to say even before I say it, Lord. You go before me and follow me. You place Your hand of blessing on my head. Such knowledge is too wonderful for me, too great for me to understand!"[3]

He knows what I'm going to say before I say it. He even helps me say it. He takes away the fear of staring into a camera, speaking into a microphone or looking out at the faces of those at a conference or workshop. These days I do all those things with ease only because I have the assurance God does know me.

I still feel my voice is loudest when I write, but there is no doubt speaking, coaching and podcasting is also a part of God's plan for the message He has given me to share with the world.

GOD LAUGHS

Oaths sworn on oak trees don't last after all. I think God set me up that day. He knew one day that scared little girl would be speaking in front of potential audiences of millions. Even now I can hear Him chuckle about this turn of events which didn't take Him by surprise at all.

For many years I had left the little girl version of me crying at the oak tree on a cold December day. She remembered she couldn't count on adults to help her when she was in a bind. She was scared, alone and embarrassed to be on stage with what seemed like the whole universe watching her colossal failure.

Although Grandma did not set me up for failure and apologized for insisting I learn one poem too many, the fear of that day was still very real. Throughout grade school, high school and college I avoided having to give any kind of speeches or oral reports. I was afraid of falling flat on my face.

To break this stronghold of I don't have a voice, God used love-filled people to help me see being in front of people could be a good experience, no matter what my size. He used a seminar filled with professionals to let me know I could actually say more than two words and make them have meaning.

He showed me transformation from a scared little girl to a self-assured adult is possible, but only when I allow Him to tear down every part of the stronghold I had set up to protect myself from being humiliated.

> God knows me. He knows what gifts I need to share the message He has put on my heart.

The little girl had experienced the fear of looking like a fool. As an adult, I knew those fears were childish, but the part of me which was afraid needed to be acknowledged, loved and accepted.

I am so glad God knows me, really knows me. He knows what gifts I need to share the message He has put on my heart. I am flooded with extreme joy, peace and thankfulness for what God has done in my life.

God does have power to break our strongholds, especially if the lies we are believing are getting in the way of what He has in store for us. The stronghold of I don't have a voice had to be broken for me to step into the destiny God had planned for me since the beginning of time.

ENDNOTES

1. Psalm 139:15-16 NLT
2. Romans 8:28 TPT
3. Psalm 139:4-6 NLT

"We are convinced that every detail of our lives is continually woven together to fit into God's perfect plan of bringing good into our lives, for we are His lovers who have been called to fulfill His designed purpose."

ROMANS 8:28 TPT

CHAPTER 13

GOD DIRECTS MY DESTINY

I always loved it when foreign missionaries came to speak at our church. They were usually scheduled for a Sunday or Wednesday night service. They brought slides with them of exotic places. They told stories of foreign mission fields where God moved in extraordinary ways. The missionaries would tell of the hardships they had moving to a foreign country, learning a new language, immersing themselves and their families in a different culture and sharing Jesus in new and creative ways.

With the emphasis on missions and my desire to do something special in God's Kingdom, it wasn't unusual I went forward in several services over the years to volunteer to be a foreign missionary. I had my heart set on helping people and at the same time telling their stories to others who might not be able to go to a foreign country, but they could help send missionaries.

I went to college on a mission's scholarship. I knew I didn't want to be a preacher or teacher. Maybe I would marry a preacher who would also be a foreign missionary? Maybe I could use my writing skills in some way? I didn't know, but I wanted to find out and I was grateful for the help of the scholarship.

FOREIGN MISSIONARY?

Right out of college I worked in the press office of a denominational foreign mission board. They had a program for college graduates to spend two years on the mission field. It seemed I was in the right place at the right time. I could go on the mission field and write news stories about the work they were doing. I was on my way to God's purpose for my life.

I prayed about it and finally got my application in barely under the deadline. It didn't take long for me to get the response letter. I had been rejected. I was slightly more than 20 percent over normal weight. The letter politely explained how being overweight can affect health issues especially when living in overseas countries. If I could lose the weight in two months, I would be accepted on a provisional basis.

I threw the letter away. I didn't think I could lose the 35 plus pounds I needed to lose before the deadline. I was miffed. I was mad at the program. I didn't want anyone to know I had been rejected because of my weight.

I decided God didn't have a destiny for me and couldn't use me in any significant way. My self-esteem was at a record low. The evil one loves to kick us when we are down. He knows all he has to do is twist the knife in further.

For years I had been looking forward to graduating from college and stepping into my calling. I was sure God would use me because I'd heard all of my life all I needed to do was be available. I'd said, "Here I am God." It felt like He said, "But you're too fat."

Still, if God wanted me to go to the mission field, He could override the decision. He could move the director of the program to pick up the phone and call me and say, "Oh I'm sorry. We didn't know it was you. Of course, we want you in our program. We'd love to have you write stories about what we're doing."

The call never came. Instead of asking God what He wanted me to do, I listened to the voice of the enemy which said, "God could never use you. You're too fat. God doesn't use fat people. He likes skinny people better. You're fat. You'll always be fat. Just accept it as a fact. God can't use you."

As I look back on this time I see if I believed God wanted me to go to the mission field, then I wouldn't have let 35 pounds get in my way. I would have at least tried to lose weight. If I had lost the weight and gotten anywhere near the goal, they would probably have let me into the program.

God had been trying to get my attention about my weight issue and how that connects to my destiny.

God had been trying to get my attention about my weight issue and how that connects to my destiny. I just didn't realize it. It would be years before I would understand the two themes which dominated my prayer life as an adult—my destiny and my weight—were very interconnected.

Even at the time I was turned down for the two-year program, I blatantly ignored the big billboard God was trying to get me to see. "Teresa, I want you to lose weight. I want you to be around to do My work." Instead, it felt like the organizers of the program were just being biased and only wanted pretty people to serve as their representatives.

I was embedding the lie deeper and deeper. The more I thought about the fact I couldn't be accepted for the program, I dismissed trying to lose weight to get in the next year. I figured it wasn't worth the effort because God just can't use me. I'm too fat.

DESTINY AND WEIGHT ISSUES

I had never thought about my destiny or purpose being connected to my weight. Even after being turned down for a missionary program, I didn't connect the dots. I knew I should lose weight, but was God really concerned about my weight? And if so, why?

Scripture is clear on this subject, but it's the sin that isn't popular to preach about from the pulpit. "Don't you realize that your body is the temple of the Holy Spirit, who lives in you and was given to you by God? You do not belong to yourself, for God bought you with a high price. So you must honor God with your body."[1]

This is a clear admonition to take care of the physical part of us. The next verse, though, really hits home. "All things are lawful for me, but not all things are profitable. All things are lawful for me, but I will not be mastered by anything. Food is for the stomach and the stomach is for food, but God will do away with both of them. Yet the body is not for immorality, but for the Lord, and the Lord is for the body."[2]

I knew these verses related to sexual immorality, but then why throw food in there? I understood that it was an illustration to get across a point about how both overindulging in food and being sexually immoral affect the body, but I wasn't exactly sure how they went together. Both harm the body. Both profane God's temple.

It made more sense when I read it in other versions. "Just because something is technically legal doesn't mean it's spiritually appropriate. If I went around doing whatever I thought I could get by with, I'd be a slave to my whims. You know the old saying, 'First you eat to live, and then you live to eat'? Well, it may be true that the body is only a temporary thing, but that's no excuse for stuffing your body with food or indulging it with sex. Since the Master honors you with a body, honor Him with your body!"[3]

We have no excuse to stuff our bodies with unhealthy food. In other words, overindulging in food is damaging our bodies which are the dwelling places for the Holy Spirit.

EXPENSIVE PURCHASE

"You were God's expensive purchase, paid for with tears of blood, so by all means, then, use your body to bring glory to God!"[4] It has taken me a long time to understand this. "I am God's expensive purchase paid for with tears of Jesus' blood." God sent His Son to die on a cross for me so I could live in a body. He showed me how to navigate this world as a spiritual being having a human existence. Eating myself into an early grave is not being grateful for what He did for me.

Earth is the testing ground where our character is built through trials and tests. My son-in-law loves strategy board games. They are the kind where the goals are to build kingdoms and survive all kinds of trials and tests to make it through and win the game.

It's the game of life we are living right now. However, we have a secret weapon to help us make it through. If we follow God's plans to get through this actual game of life, we will each win the crown of glory.

"My fellow believers, when it seems as though you are facing nothing, but difficulties see it as an invaluable opportunity to experience the greatest joy that you can! For you know that when your faith is tested it stirs up power within you to endure all things. And then as your endurance grows even stronger it will release perfection into every part of your being until there is nothing missing and nothing lacking."[5]

We aren't thinking about how our choices affect our purposes.

Part of the difficulties or trials and tests we are facing involves our overindulgence in certain foods. If we aren't careful this can become what we are living for. However, God wants us to understand that our lives are more than earthly and sensual indulgences. When we focus on our cravings and desires, we are trading in our eternal destinies for a bowl of stew, like Esau did.[6] It becomes all about what we want in the moment.

We aren't thinking about how our choices affect our purposes. We have gotten to the point where eternity is wrapped up in pleasing our appetites and making sure we have all the food we want.

This is where I was when I was trying to do the work God wanted me to but was also gaining weight. I wanted to follow God, but I wanted to follow Him and eat whatever I wanted. I was working hard for Him and thought I needed a reward at the end of a long day.

Whenever I get to the point where I feel like I'm working hard for God and want to reach for something I know will not benefit my body, I am no longer working for God. I am working for me. I am building my kingdom, not God's.

DESTINY DIDN'T PASS ME BY

I'll be honest. When I started my weight loss journey, it wasn't because I wanted to honor God with my body. It was because I was sick and tired of being fat and lazy. I hated what I had become. I felt God's destiny had passed me by.

From the time I was a child, a dream of mine was to write a book about someone who had done something great with God's help, something which really mattered and something which would help others. I realized I couldn't write a book when I was super morbidly obese. I had no energy, stamina, focus or clarity. I knew if I lost weight, I would be better able to write a book, but I had put writing books in the impossible category, just like losing weight.

Then losing weight and writing a book came together. I just never thought the book or books I would write one day would be about me. Once *Sweet Grace: How I Lost 250 Pounds* was published and I began teaching it at my church, I started to see how writing the story of my weight loss journey was the start of my true life's purpose. The book led to coaching others in online groups, courses and even one-on-one coaching. This was never on my radar, but it was on God's.

I went to the very first Release the Writer Workshop in March 2013 and met Wendy. After the workshop, I had a session with her. She asked me, "What do you want this book to do for you?"

I said, "What do you mean? I just know God called me to write a book. If it only helps one person, it will be enough."

Leaning in, she said, "People write books for different reasons. Some want to promote a business, become a coach, start a public speaking career or launch editing or writing services."

I thought about it for a minute. "Maybe one day I might want to help others write books, but becoming an author is enough for me."

She sat back and said, "Well, that's good for starters, but you have coaching in your future and a lot more. There are things I sense God is holding back until you are ready to hear them."

I didn't believe her, but I heard her. God made sure of that and I have not forgotten what she said. There have been days I have been so glad God didn't tell me more than I could handle. He let her tell me the first thing and that was enough of a challenge.

TELEVISION CAN BE SCARY

When I was asked to go on my first national television interview, I was scared spitless because it was a 30-minute program. I didn't know if I could do a 30-minute program. Then I was invited for a five-minute segment on a secular station with a more limited audience and decided I'd try that. I prayed hard to have the right words to answer the questions. Five minutes flew by and I knew I could have talked for 30 more.

After that short exposure, it didn't bother me to go on television talk shows and even answer tough questions. One I remember was, "I see all these shows with 500-pound people who are housebound. They have to have spouses, friends or children who are enabling them by bringing them food. Who enabled you?"

If I always tell the truth, it will always be the right answer.

I didn't miss a beat. I said, "No one enabled me. I enabled myself. At 430 pounds I could still drive and work. I went to the grocery store, shopped and cooked for my family. I just ate whatever I wanted. I needed no encouragement."

I quickly found I wasn't afraid of hard questions. If I always tell the truth, it will always be the right answer. I also know and have experienced a quick prayer and the Holy Spirit will give me the words to say when I don't have any.

All I wanted to do was write one book. Now I've written six books and two study guides. I know there will be more because I can't stop, but I never imagined all of the things which have happened. They never would have if I hadn't been obedient to finally let God lead me to do the difficult work of saying, "No" to the foods I craved, and "Yes" to the forever lifestyle change God had in store for me.

It wasn't just what I was eating and how I was moving which had to change. The biggest thing was surrendering my wants for His and giving over control of my life completely to Him.

Years ago, I thought I was doing that, but as long as I was making my appetite, desires and cravings my priority, I still had one huge area I needed to surrender to Him. I held on to sugar with tightly clenched fists daring God to pry it out of my hands, but God will never do that. He won't take from us what we are not willing to surrender to Him.

We can take it to an early grave with us, but He will not violate our free will. He gave us choices so we would willingly choose to love Him. Our love for Him is shown in how we follow and obey Him.

Will He beat us up and condemn us if we don't follow Him? No, He will not. When we finally repent of what we have done and submit completely to Him, He will welcome us with open arms. Then, He will begin to trust us with the plans He has for us.

> Our surrender to Him must come before we step into our purpose.

"Out of our surrender to Christ suddenly there is the discovery of purpose," Bill Johnson, said. I know the truth of this now, but I didn't know it when I was struggling for years unwilling to surrender sugar and comfort foods to Him.

God won't move us towards our purpose until we have surrendered everything to Him. We must hold everything loosely and willingly let go when He asks us to. If there is even one thing we are holding back from Him, we are not ready to step into our purpose. He won't trust us with what He has for us until we trust Him with everything we are clinging to so tightly. Our surrender to Him must come before we step into our purpose.

God had a plan for my life. He knew exactly what I had to do before I could step into His plan. He didn't lay it all out for me. He just asked me to follow Him each step of the way. I didn't get very far until I balked like a stubborn Missouri mule. Weight loss and my destiny were interwoven, but the foods I loved were what I couldn't seem to surrender. Until I surrendered them, God couldn't show me the next step in my destiny.

I see all through my life how He prepared me for what He wanted me to do. My education, courses I took, certifications I got, the information I garnered and the strongholds He helped me break all prepared me for the time when I would be thrust into a destiny I never dreamed was possible.

> Weight loss and my destiny were interwoven, but the foods I loved were what I couldn't surrender.

I shouldn't have doubted He had a destiny and a purpose for me, though. He tells me plainly He does. "We have become His poetry, a re-created people that will fulfill the destiny He has given each of us, for we are joined to Jesus, the Anointed One. Even before we were born, God planned in advance our destiny and the good works we would do to fulfill it!"[7]

God is more concerned about us fulfilling our destinies than we are. He knows who we are. He knows how we will mess up His plans, but He still helps us get back on the right path headed towards our destiny with purpose and determination to follow Him every step of the way.

As much as we love sugar and comfort foods now, it can never compare with the sweetness following Him provides when we finally surrender everything to Him. "When God fulfills your longings, sweetness fills your soul."[8]

I love knowing I am headed in the direction He has for me. For years I tried to figure things out on my own and make them happen. All along God was trying to help me understand how to follow Him in all things. The biggest area of disobedience I had was running to foods made with processed sugar for my comfort and protection.

God knew if I would listen to Him and allow Him to help me break the strongholds keeping me bound in sugar addiction, it would be a sweet surrender to Him. Nothing would hold me back once I was all in with Him.

God wants us to fall head over heels in ove with Him.

He desires we choose Him above all the noise of this world, above all the noise of those around us, above all the noise in our heads. He wants us to fall head over heels in love with Him. He will know when we are there because we will hold nothing back. When we surrender it all to Him, suddenly things will begin to happen we never in a million years imagined. He will catapult us toward our purpose.

He has been working with us since before we were born. Our destiny is wrapped up and tied with a bow, a beautiful gift to us. All we have to do is surrender everything to Him.

In the seconds it takes us to pray a prayer of total and complete surrender withholding nothing from Him, our lives can drastically change. It's time. He's calling.

What will your answer be?

ENDNOTES

1. 1 Cor 6:19-20 NLT
2. 1 Cor 6:12 NASB
3. 1 Cor. 6:19-20 MSG
4. 1 Cor. 6:19-20 TPT
5. James 1:2-4 TPT
6. Genesis 25:29-34 NIV
7. Ephesians 2:10 TPT
8. Proverbs 13:19 TPT

*"We have become His
poetry, a re-created people
that will fulfill the destiny
He has given each of us,
for we are joined to Jesus,
the Anointed One. Even
before we were born, God
planned in advance our
destiny and the good works
we would do to fulfill it!"*

EPHESIANS 2:10 TPT

CHAPTER 14

I TRUST YOU JESUS

I was a sophomore in college when my dorm father asked me to tutor a Chinese girl who lived down the hall from me. May was thin and graceful. Our tutoring sessions consisted of walking the campus and talking about the history we Americans take for granted.

I took this frail and beautiful Chinese freshman under my wing. A quiet, peaceful young lady, she would ask me questions she was too shy to ask in class. She was bright and loved being able just to talk with someone who would take time to listen and understand her questions.

We had been working together for a couple of months when she started having severe headaches. Her aunt flew her to California for treatment. A few days later, my beautiful friend died of a brain aneurysm.

Her death hit me hard. She was my same age and a Christian. One day she was alive. The next day, she was gone but where did she go? And where would I go when I died? Was there a heaven? If so, how did I know for sure I'd go there when I died?

I lay awake at night watching the flames rise in the gas heater in my dorm room. They reminded me of everything I had been told about hell. I didn't dare go to sleep. I could believe ardently in hell, but heaven seemed to be more of a leap of faith than I could make.

At the age of seven, I had accepted Christ as my Savior mainly to avoid those dreaded flames. Now they seemed to be right in the room with me. Having grown up in church, I'd heard plenty of hell-fire and brimstone messages. I knew what the scriptures said.

What I wanted, though, was hard and fast evidence that when I died, I'd go to heaven. I know there's a moon because a man walked on it and brought back a moon rock. Plus, I could see it up in the sky, but how did I know for sure there was heaven?

When I asked people on campus, they all gave me Bible verses to prove the existence of heaven, streets of gold, pearly gates, city four-square. It was nothing new to me. "I know that already," I wanted to scream at them. Give me real, solid, hold-in-my-hands evidence.

IS HEAVEN REAL?

I was exhausted having gotten no answers to my questions and very little sleep. I wanted and needed answers. I knew only one person I could trust to give me an honest answer and thankfully I was going home for Thanksgiving. My dad had always told me the truth. I was desperate to talk to him. It felt like my entire life depended on it.

The minute I got home, I grabbed him and sat him down at the kitchen table. "Dad, can you give me tangible, irrefutable proof that there is a heaven?" Instead of giving me an instant pat answer, he thought through his answer before speaking.

"I know what you want," he said, "but I can't give you the evidence you can hold in your hand. Some claim they have gone to heaven and have come back but that's just their word. It's not provable because it can't be validated. I can't travel there and prove heaven exists and come back here and tell you."

> Can you give me tangiible, irrefutable proof that there is a heaven?

He continued to explain what he could tell me was that the Bible says there is a heaven. It says those who believe, trust, rely on and live their lives for Jesus Christ will go there when they die. He reminded me that Jesus was indeed a living, breathing person who was resurrected from the dead and seen by more than 500 people.

He held up his worn Bible and said, "I choose to believe the words of this book. If when I die there is not a heaven, I will have at least lived my life for a purpose greater than me. It's a decision that's much more than just being saved from the flames of hell."

What he said struck a chord deep within me. His answer was honest. "One more thing," he added, "you can't just decide you're going to believe what the Bible says about heaven and ignore everything else it says. When you believe one part, you have to believe it all. Live your life based on this book and you'll have a real reason to live."

He took my hand, looked me in the eyes and said, "Trust in Jesus. Surrender completely to Him and He will never fail you." Before that minute, I didn't realize I had a trust issue, but right then I realized I did. I had resisted surrendering completely to Jesus on the slim chance there wasn't a heaven. It was what I was looking for.

Strongholds are what we trust instead of trusting God.

Recently I was reminded of Dad's admonition when I heard the explanation that strongholds are what we trust instead of trusting in God. Back in college, I had been afraid to put all my eggs in God's basket. As such, I was pretty much going crazy because I didn't know what or who to trust. I didn't want to trust in the world. Still, it took a huge leap of faith for me to finally put my entire life and future in God's hands.

God doesn't want to be at the top of my list, He wants to be my list period. Nothing should exist on my to-do list unless it goes through the filter of what Jesus wants for my life. I shouldn't be the director and orchestrator of my life. I have surrendered those positions to Jesus.

It's a faith issue. It's a trust issue. It's a total surrender issue.

TRUSTING GOD

It reminds me of the story where King Asa of Judah didn't rely on God to help him. He relied on the king of Syria instead. The Prophet Hanani told King Asa, "The eyes of the Lord search the whole earth in order to strengthen those whose hearts are fully committed to Him. What a fool you have been! From now on you will be at war."[1] King Asa chose wrongly and five years later he died.

God is telling us if we trust in Him with all that is within us, He will keep strengthening us. He will continue to help us because we have put Him first, but if we don't His protection is lifted. What a scary thing.

The lies we believe don't scream at us. Instead, they whisper softly, just like they did to King Asa. He wanted some physical proof that he would be protected. That's why he relied on the King of Syria instead of God. It's exactly what I was asking for when I wanted proof that there is a heaven. Instead, Dad helped me understand that trusting Jesus is like taking a leap of faith.

> The lies we believe don't scream at us—they whisper softly.

The hard thing about a leap of faith is that we first have to jump and then trust God that where we land will be right in the middle of His grace. One thing I know, if we never take that leap, we will never experience His grace. We will be stuck in our humanity and never experience the sovereign majesty and power of our supernatural God.

We can't understand it because we are human, natural, fleshly, soulish in nature. Jesus tells us, though, that without trusting in Him we will always and forever be stuck. Trusting Jesus frees us.

Jesus said to the Jews who were claiming to believe Him, "If you stick with this, living out what I tell you, you are my disciples for sure. Then you will experience for yourselves the truth, and the truth will free you."[2]

When they argued with Him saying they had never been slaves to anyone, so they didn't need to be free, He explained that He was coming from a different perspective than they were. They were thinking in physical terms of being a slave. He was speaking in spiritual terms.

"'I speak eternal truth,' Jesus said. 'When you sin you are not free. You've become a slave in bondage to your sin. And slaves have no permanent standing in a family, like a son does, for a son is a part of the family forever. So if the Son sets you free from sin, then become a true son and be unquestionably free!'"[3]

Lies appear to be true to us because we look at them from our limited perspective. The Jews were looking through an earthly lens. Jesus, though, had an entirely different perspective. He was trying to help them to see that there is more to life than the physical world we live in. Freedom is a spiritual mindset. If we could only tap into that on our journeys, what a difference it would make.

WHOLE, HEALTHY, HAPPY

In 1994, I got a little taste of how to do that. During Freedom Seminar, I made a contract with myself. Everyone in the group was challenged to think about what we wanted to accomplish in life. At that time the biggest thing I wanted was to write a book about someone who did something that mattered. I knew God had shown me I would one day write a book like this. However, every time I thought I had gotten close to doing it something had fallen through.

One woman I worked with and interviewed for weeks filling endless stacks of cassette tapes decided she didn't want to do the book unless it could be a nonfiction book. I had told her at the outset that since her story involved a lot of allegations, I wouldn't do the book unless we did it as fiction based on fact. I had to back out of the process and get a lawyer involved.

God protected me from what could have been a disaster. Still, I knew He had called me to write a book. I just didn't know what book it would be.

It dared me to go deep in order to find out what God wanted me to belive was possible for my life.

To get in touch with what God wanted for our lives, we were asked to choose words to define what attributes would a person have to have who could do what we wanted to do. It's difficult to describe the intensity of this session. It was a defining moment. It dared me to go deep in order to find out what God wanted me to believe was possible for my life.

At the time I weighed probably over 400 pounds. I was tired, lethargic, had no stamina or energy. I could barely walk. Everything hurt. My brain was foggy and I couldn't think clearly. In other words, I was far from being able to stay with a book-length project.

More than anything else, I wanted to be holy. During a training session, Russ had defined the word "holy" as whole and healthy. That really resonated with me but messed with my definition of holy as being sacred or set apart. It does mean that, but Russ was explaining what it means for a human being to be holy. That's an entirely different ballgame.

According to an online search, the English origin of the word holy dates back to the 11th century and comes from the Old

English word halig, which is an adjective derived from the hal which means whole. The Scottish hale of "health, happiness and wholeness" is the most complete form of this Old Engish root word. This defines exactly what I wanted my life to be.

To be whole means I need to be complete in every part of me—body, soul and spirit. At the time, I felt my body was the most incomplete part of me. I could not be a whole person if my body was barely hanging together. My soul, or my mind, will and emotions, had some issues as well.

> To be whole means I need to be complete in every part of me— body, soul and spirit.

As long as my spirit was aligned with God's Spirit, I felt I was doing alright, but I saw my spirit was not fully aligned with God's. I didn't want what God wanted for me. I wasn't trusting Him to lead me. I was trusting myself. I was bound and determined to eat what I wanted whenever I wanted no matter what God said. I was not being Spirit-led at all. The biggest issue on my weight loss journey was that I did not trust God even though I thought I had fixed that years ago.

I had to be healthy in all of those areas to be whole and I wasn't. I was lacking in every area. Without being whole and healthy I could not begin to write a book. It would be impossible.

Another thing I was sadly lacking was joy. I needed the joy of the Lord to be my strength. I couldn't continue to go around in an almost drugged state, which was caused by the types of foods I couldn't stop eating. Joy didn't go with my other two words, so I chose the word happy, which does align better with the Scottish meaning of that adjective.

What type of woman could write a book that mattered? A whole, healthy, happy woman. In 1994, weighing at least 400 pounds, I declared before a seminar of at least 30 people that I am a whole, healthy, happy woman. At that time just looking at me, one could tell I was far from that.

Every time I met with a group of people from my seminar, they would ask me, "Who are you?" I would answer, "I am a whole, healthy, happy woman." I still weighed over 400 pounds when I was saying that. Was it the truth or a lie?

It was a prophecy. It was how I defined myself because I knew it was what God wanted for me. Even when I started defining myself this way, I didn't believe anything would happen to change me. Eventually, though, God helped me step into the truth that He defined for me. That only happened as I began to learn to trust Him and not the lies I believed.

I had to dispel the lies like I'm fat and will always be fat, I can never lose weight, even God can't help me lose weight, and all the others I had believed that had become strongholds in my life. Then I had to accept and believe God's truth. Doing that changed me and I lost over 250 pounds. It wasn't easy. It wasn't quick. It was a total lifestyle change. I am different only because I have learned to take that leap of faith and trust Jesus with every part of me.

> It was a prophecy. It was how I defined myself because I knew it was what God wanted for me.

There are always challenges when we live changed lives. Paul talks about it in these pivotal scriptures. "For though we live in the world, we do not wage war as the world does. The weapons we fight with are not the weapons of the world. On the contrary, they have divine power to demolish strongholds. We demolish arguments and every pretension that sets itself up against the knowledge of God, and we take captive every thought to make it obedient to Christ."[4]

Incorrect thinking empowers the enemy.

When we are trying to live changed lives, we must change our thinking because our incorrect thinking empowers the enemy. What defines incorrect thinking? It is an argument or idea that goes against the knowledge of God. Most of us know who God is. We have correct theology.

If someone said to us, "Do you believe God can do anything?" We'd say yes. We know God is all-powerful, all-present, all-knowing. Of course, we believe He can do anything. However, when it comes to our lives, we waiver. Can He heal me? Can He heal my child? Can He help me lose the weight I need to lose? Can He get me out of debt? Can He save my marriage?

It's not knowledge that we have a problem with, it's our thoughts that form a lifestyle that goes against the very thing we say we believe. We have a problem between facts and implementation or active reliance on what we say we believe. This is a lifestyle problem.

One bad thought or one lie isn't necessarily a stronghold. However, if we don't take that thought captive, it will become a stronghold. It will grow because we will continue to feed it. This is true especially if we don't give God room to work and bring about what only He can accomplish. We don't understand how God can do what looks impossible, so we choose not to put our trust in Him completely. By doing so we leave a place for the enemy to invade and hide in a stronghold we created for Him.

On Sunday morning we say we trust Him, but the rest of the week we make excuses for Him which allows the enemy to work all the harder on us. We may even decide that we can handle things better than God, so we try to fix the issue. All that does is delay the time when God can work on our problem. When we're in the way, He stays out of the way.

TAKING THOUGHTS CAPTIVE

Once we see and understand what we have been doing we have to take those thoughts captive. We recognize what the thought is. This is key because we've given it a place to hide. It doesn't like to be exposed. Once we realize what lies we are believing, we must write them down.

Recently I had surgery. One lie I believed before the surgery was, "The surgeons don't know what to do and even God can't help them and me. This won't work." I wrote that down. Then I wrote down what I knew was true as I partnered with God. "I don't understand how this physical issue will be fixed, but I trust You, God. When no one else can help me, Jesus can."

I trust You, God. When no one else can help me, Jesus can.

I recognized the fallacy was a stronghold that was keeping me from even deciding to have the surgery. Then I partnered with God to trust Him. I have to admit, I was scared and I shed quite a few tears. However, when I started repeating the truth over and over again, the fear left. I was able to go forward and make some rational decisions based on what I know God wanted for me which is to be restored, renewed and revived.

Strongholds are thought patterns that begin to invade our lifestyle. They seep in slowly and before we know it, we are no longer believing the truth about God. We are believing lies. What we must do is take command over those lies and tell the devil, "This lie stops here."

Strongholds are things in which we trust. That means they are also things in which others trust. This can include individuals, families, areas or cities. We can help others overcome their strongholds when we allow God to break ours. Proverbs says, "A wise man scales the city of the mighty and brings down the stronghold in which they trust."[5]

The wise man or wise woman is someone who has conquered their strongholds and put their trust where it belongs which is in God completely. When they have done that, they can help pull down others' strongholds. It still takes their cooperation with God to get it done, but they can help by interceding for them.

RESULTS OF TRUSTING JESUS

Remember the prophetic declaration I made? Today I can say as a testimony to my God, "I am a whole, healthy, happy woman." In follow-up sessions, I added to that. Take into consideration that when I added this to my prophetic declaration, I still hadn't written even one book.

The entire statement with the addition says, "I am a whole, healthy, happy woman of God administering grace and truth in a powerful way energized by the power of the Holy Spirit." That statement defines who I am today.

It's about more than losing weight. It's about trusting Jesus with every fiber of my being. In the process, many great things have happened not the least of which has been writing this book. I love my life and I love knowing I finally have my trust where it needs to be. I trust You, Jesus.

The book of Nahum tells us, "The Lord is good, a stronghold in the day of trouble; And He knows those who trust in Him."[6] Trusting God is at the core of everything regarding our spiritual journeys. We definitely want God to be our stronghold. We do that by trusting only in Him and not in anything else.

We definitely want God to be our stronghold.

I'm so glad Dad helped me as a crazy college student to place all my trust in Jesus. I am more awash in the Holy Spirit today. I have the peace of God which surpasses all understanding and is guarding my heart and mind in Christ Jesus.[7] It's impossible to explain because it goes beyond natural understanding. It can only be described as supernatural.

I know many don't have this peace and that makes me sad. We can have God's peace by simply putting all our trust in His Son, Jesus. I envision it like I have a huge basket and a lot of eggs. They all go in the Jesus basket with nothing left over to put anywhere else.

It's a surrender issue. It's a trust issue.

I trust You, Jesus.

ENDNOTES

1. 2 Chronicles 16:9 NLT
2. John 8:31-32 MSG
3. John 8:34-36 TPT
4. 2 Corinthians 10:3-5 NIV
5. Proverbs 21:22 NASB
6. Nahum 1:7-8 NKJV
7. Philippians 4:7 NKJV

ACTION STEPS

CHAPTER 1: MY STRENGTH COMES FROM GOD

Lie: I'm not strong enough to give up sugar

Truth: My strength comes from God.

Journal your answers to these and questions in other sections.

1. What foods are you eating when you eat unhealthily or what habits? List all that cause you problems.

2. When are you most prone to do this?
   What's happening at that time t?

3. Do you feel like you can't stop or is it that you don't want to stop?

4. What thoughts go through your mind when you are doing this?

5. Do you feel you are weak around certain foods or substances and can't say no? List those. What can you do to not give in?

6. In what way can seeing yourself as weak help you? See 2 Cor. 12:9-10 AMP.

7. What is holding you back from activating the dynamic power of the Holy Spirit in your life?

CHAPTER 2: GOD IS MY GOD

Lie: My stomach my god.

Truth: God is my God

1. What lie do you believe and how is that holding you back from following God completely?

2. How does this lie affect your relationship with God?

3. What's God's secret truth He is revealing to you?

4. What do you need to surrender to God? When will you do that?

5. "When I do what I know He's asking me to do, then and only then have I correctly chosen life. My actions reveal my choice." What do you have to change to really show God you are choosing life?

6. Will you commit to change that this week? It may mean committing to learning how to step away from a bad habit you know God doesn't like. It may mean doing something God has placed on your heart. Be specific.

7. Have you placed something or someone on the throne of your life other than God? Is that thing or person more important than God? It's time to take that thing or person off the throne and put God there. Will you do that today?

CHAPTER 3: WITH GOD ALL THINGS ARE POSSIBLE

Lie: Losing weight is impossible for me.

Truth: With God all things are possible.

1. What have been your experiences with losing weight? List the major diets or plans you've been on and what happened.

2. Did you lose weight or not?

3. If you lost weight, even initially, what worked to help you lose weight?

4. If you lost and gained weight back, what happened to cause you to gain the weight back?

5. Maybe there is a different bad habit or addiction that you have placed in the category of being impossible to give up. Go through this same process only thinking about the times you tried and failed to give this up. Make a list of those times and what you did and why it failed.

6. Read Luke 18:27. Do you believe God can do the impossible in your life where weight is concerned? Why or why not?

7. What would daily living in the Spirit look like regarding your healthy living journey?

CHAPTER 4: GOD DOES NOT CONDEMN MY FAILURE

Lie: I am a failure.

Truth: God does not condemn my failure.

1. Do you feel like a failure? Where do you feel you have failed?

2. Are there any things you feel guilty about? List those.

3. Have you asked God to forgive you for those things? If not do that now.

4. Do you feel shame and condemnation for what you did? If yes, do you feel like God has forgiven you? If not, read 1 John 1:9 and ask Him again to forgive you.

5. Then, tell God that you choose to forgive yourself. Take the step of actually forgiving yourself now.

6. I had to choose to forgive the third grader even though I was an adult. I just said to Jesus, "I choose to forgive him for calling me a four-eyed fatso. I renounce the lie that You see me as fat. What is Your truth?" He poured His truth over me. I did the same regarding the college boys even though I didn't know who they were. If you still feel shame and condemnation, ask God to show you the root of that. If it is a specific situation, forgive those who had a part in it. Journal your thoughts.

7. It's amazing how freeing it can be to forgive, to renounce the lie that we believe God is saying the same thing about us, and to hear His truth. He never condemns. He always redeems. In what way has He redeemed some of your failures?

CHAPTER 5: JESUS WANTS ME TO FOLLOW HIM

Lie: I have to follow the rules to be a good Christian.

Truth: Jesus wants me to follow Him.

1. What rules did you feel obligated to follow to be a good Christian?

2. Whose rules were they?

3. How did you feel if you broke the rules?

4. If you didn't grow up in the church or with a family who gave you rules, how did not having rules make you feel?

5. How have rules regarding dealing with the opposite sex either helped or hurt you?

6. What does it mean to you to be saved by grace and not by the law, rules or works?

7. What does it look like to follow Jesus instead of rules?

CHAPTER 6: GOD IS MY PROTECTOR

Lie: I have to self-protect.

Truth: God is my Protector.

1. What or whom are you afraid of?

2. Have you forgiven them by just stating to God that you forgive them and renouncing the lie that God will not protect you? If not, do that now.

3. After doing that, ask God, "What is your truth?" He will answer you. Don't force the answer. It will be the first thing you think, see or sense after you ask Him. Write down what happened.

4. If you don't understand His answer, ask Him. God loves to answer our questions.

5. What do you do to protect yourself? How has that worked for you?

6. How does it make you feel to always be afraid and have to protect yourself?

7. Read Psalm 91. List all of God's promises in this chapter. Claim them as yours by putting your name in the chapter. Here's an example from verse 1 that says: Those who live in the shelter of the Most High will find rest in the shadow of the Almighty.

I rewrote it to say: "Because Teresa lives in the shelter of the Most High, I will find rest in the shadow of the Almighty."

Do that using your name with the rest of the chapter. Read it to yourself each morning until it becomes truth to you.

.

CHAPTER 7: I MATTER TO GOD

Lie: I don't matter to my mother.
Truth: I matter to God.

1. Do you feel like you matter? I hope you do, but if you don't, what makes you think you don't matter?

2. Who in your life do you feel you do not matter to?

3. What specific incidents make you think that?

4. How did that affect you as a child?

5. Can you see how that is still impacting you as an adult?

6. If you remember the specific circumstance, try saying to God, I chose to forgive (the person) for what they did or said. I renounce the lie that God will treat me that same way. Then, ask Him what His truth is. He will tell you. It may be in the form of a thought, feeling or words. Be sure to write His truth down and ask Him more if it is not clear to you. God loves to answer our questions.

7. Do you feel that you matter to God? Look up the scriptures below and write down what they tell you about how you matter to God.

- Romans 5:8

- John 16:33

- 2 Peter 5:7

- Joshua 1:9

- Isaiah 41:10

- Philippians 4:19

- Psalm 119:114

- Psalm 23:3

- Isaiah 30:21

- Zephaniah 3:17

CHAPTER 8: GOD VALUES ME FOR ME

Lie: I Am Only Valuable for What I Do

Truth: God Values Me for Me

1. What are some words that define your life's mission?

2. Read Psalms 139 NLT. What does this tell you about why God created you?

3. Read Ephesians 1:11-12 MSG. Where do we find our purpose?

4. Read Romans 8:28 TPT. What does God say about the timeline of your purpose?

5. Who does God say you are?

6. Do you work at a career or profession? Who would you be without that career?

7. Who are you? What are some of your positive attributes that don't relate to what you do?

CHAPTER 9: GOD WILL HELP ME

Lie: I hate exercise.

Truth: God will help me.

1. What types of exercise or play did you do as a child? Did you enjoy any sports? If you did, why did you stop?

2. How do you feel about exercise now?

3. Read 1 Cor. 6:19-20 In what way does this challenge you?

4. Read Hebrews 12:1-2 NIV. What does this say to you about your journey?

5. Read Hebrews 12:12-13 NIV. On the days I think I can't possibly go on, He tells me to:

6. Is there any exercise you enjoy now or think you might enjoy? Draw a line through those you dislike or don't want to try. Circle those you would like to try. Star those you will do.
   - Walking
   - Jogging
   - Weight training
   - Stationary bikes
   - Ice skating
   - Dancing
   - Aerobics
   - Exercise videos

- Yoga
- Bike riding
- Roller Skating
- Treadmill
- Swimming
- Water jogging
- Jump Rope
- Trampoline
- Walking your Dog
- Zumba
- Water aerobics
- Team sports
- Rollerblading
- Skiing
- Triathlon
- 5K
- Sky diving
- Parasailing
- Surf boarding

7. Which exercise will you begin this week?

CHAPTER 10: GOD ANSWERS MY PRAYERS

Lie: God doesn't answer my prayers.

Truth: God answers my prayers.

1. When has there been a time you felt God didn't hear or answer your prayer?

2. What was the reason you felt He didn't answer it? Was it because He didn't answer it in your timeframe? Was it because He didn't answer it how you wanted it answered? Was it because He said, "No?" Was it because He said, "Yes?"

3. If it wasn't answered in the way you wanted, what did that make you think?

4. What does 1 John 5:14-15 tell you about prayer?

5. How do these verses change the way you understand prayer?

6. What is the most important ingredient to you in answered prayer?

7. For more on prayer, look up the following scriptures. Draw a line from the central theme to the scripture.

SCRIPTURES

- Matthew 21:21-22
- Matthew 7:7-8
- Psalms 40:1
- John 15:7
- Psalm 66:19
- Mark 11:24

THEME

- Believe
- Keep Asking
- God Listens
- Ask in Faith
- God Helps Me
- Abide in Jesus

CHAPTER 11: HOLY SPIRIT IS MY COMFORTER

Lie: I get my comfort from the food Grandma cooked.

Truth: Holy Spirit is my Comforter.

1. How has food been used as a comfort for you? What types of food? Who prepared it?

2. What foods do you turn to for comfort? Or what other things do you turn to?

3. How do these foods comfort you?

4. Do they really provide lasting comfort?

5. How are they uncomfortable to you?

6. Read John 14: 16-18. What is one major attribute of the Holy Spirit?

7. How can the Holy Spirit bring you even better comfort than comfort foods?

CHAPTER 12: GOD KNOWS ME

Lie: I don't have a voice.

Truth: God knows me.

1. Describe a time when you failed at something and you were afraid to try it again.

2. How has that impacted your life?

3. In what ways has God led you to try to overcome that?

4. What is one gift or talent that you think you are lacking, but if you had that gift or talent God could use it to help you fulfill your purpose? Have you talked to God about that?

5. What is a dream that you have?

6. What would be one step you could take towards that dream? Could you take a course, go to a seminar, read a book, set up a website?

7. Write 300-500 words on your life manifesto. Include at least one scripture. Share it with someone. Start with My life mission is ….

CHAPTER 13: GOD DIRECTS MY DESTINY

Lie: God Can't Use Me

Truth: God Directs My Destiny

1. What are you holding on to with tightly clenched fists daring God to pry out of your hand?

2. Why are you afraid to surrender this to God?

3. What will it take for you to willingly surrender this to God so you can begin your true destiny journey in Him?

4. What is a dream you have of what you might be able to do but feel unable to do right now? Write about what would happen if you surrendered to God the things you think you can't do without?

5. What could God do with one life totally surrendered to Him?

6. What could He do with your life it was totally surrendered to Him?

7. What would it take for you to surrender your life totally to Him?

CHAPTER 14—I TRUST YOU, JESUS

Lie: I Trust In Me

Truth: I Trust You, Jesus

1. If your trust in Jesus was registered on a scale of 0 to 10, where would it fall? 0 is I don't trust Jesus with my life. 10 is I trust Jesus with every aspect of my life. Journal about why you chose that number. If it is less than 10, what would it take to make it a 10?

2. Read 2 Chronicles 16:9 NLT. What does this say to you about your trust level?

3. What would be your prophetic declaration about what kind of person God wants you to be? Choose words that describe the type of person that could do the things God has placed in your heart for you to accomplish.

4. In what way is your theology or beliefs misaligned with how you are living your life?

5. How can you take a thought captive? Write down a lie you are believing right now. Below it write the truth that God wants you to believe. Put the truth somewhere you see it often. Repeat it over and over to yourself until you replace the lie you believe with God's truth.

6. Read Nahum 1:7-8. Why is this central to our total lifestyle change and spiritual journey?

7. Have you completely surrendered to Jesus? Is there anything you are holding back just for you? Imagine you have two baskets and 10 eggs. Now actually find two containers. Mark one Jesus and one with your name.Next cut our 10 or more egg shapes out of a piece of paper. Label each of these 10 eggs with the things that matter most in your life. That could be a person, thing, issue, situation, desire or whatever God is showing you.

Now, one at a time take each one and put in the container that indicates who you are trusting to take care of that person, issue, situation or desire.. If you need to make more eggs an add more items to your containers do that. If specific foods are an issue for you, be sure you have an egg for that.

If you have anything in the basket with your name on it, ask God why you can't trust Jesus with that? What is standing in the way of you letting go of this completely? Ask Him to show what the withhold is that you have regarding this thing.

Then deal with it in the way God shows you. When you are ready, move it to the other basket. Keep these nearby so they can remind you of what issues you have trusted to Jesus and what issues you still need to release to Him.

This is a great exercise to show you where your trust level really is. It will show you the areas you still need to surrender to God. Remember, this journey of breaking strongholds is at its core, a trust and surrender issue.

It starts right here with trusting God with that problem you've been trying to fix on your own. He longs to help you. Let Him.

NEXT STEPS

Sweet Surrender was born out of my personal heartaches and victories. Your surrender will be birthed in yours as well. Don't be dismayed, though, because I have even more resources to help. On my website, you can access my coaching group, one-on-one coaching, podcast episodes, blogs and books. There are some free resources as well.

By far, my best resource is Overcomers Christian Weight Loss Coaching Academy. We have a guided experience through my extensive video course library. We also have monthly live video calls and a private Facebook group for connection. The information and signup page is on my website under the weight loss tab.

FREE GIFTS FOR MY READERS

Just for the readers of this book, I've designed scripture cards with some of the verses you just read. You can download them, print them out and use them to memorize verses. Or print them out on cards and mail to friends with an encouraging word.

The private link is just for you, my reader. You won't find it anywhere else except in this book. Copy this link: https://teresashieldsparker.com/gift/. Then, put it in your browser, share your email with us and download your gorgeous cards. You'll also get news and other information from us from time to time.

If you haven't discovered it already, I have a free ebook called "What Is A Stronghold?" This gives my explanation of what strongholds are, where they originate and how Satan uses them against God's people. Find it under the free tab on my website.

This is material I wrote when I was first researching information about strongholds. I left it out of this book, but it is good information you will find helpful. There are also some Action Steps which help personalize it for you. It's a way to introduce others to the concepts in this book.

By the way, *Sweet Surrender: Breaking Strongholds* would be a great book to use for small group study or a book club discussion group. Just use the Action Steps as talking points. You can include the ebook as an information session to introduce the book study. If you do study this book in a group, please drop me an email or find me on social media and let me know. I love to hear how people are using my books.

As always, I'd love to connect with you on any of my social media channels. I do enjoy hearing from readers. Feel free to contact me by email with questions or insights. You can find me everywhere. And thanks in advance for writing a review on Amazon. You rock!

Don't forget to download your beautiful 4-color Scripture cards as my gift to you!

LET'S CONNECT

WEBSITE	https://TeresaShieldsParker.com
AMAZON	https://amazon.com/author/ teresashieldsparker/
PODCAST	https://TeresaShieldsParker.com/Podcast/
YOUTUBE	https://youtube.com/teresashieldsparker1
FACEBOOK	https://www.facebook.com/ TeresaShieldsParker
INSTAGRAM	https://www.instagram.com/treeparker/
PINTEREST	https://www.pinterest.com/treeparker/
EMAIL	info@TeresaShieldsParker.com

Don't Forget to
DOWNLOAD YOUR FREE SCRIPTURE CARDS HERE:
HTTPS://TERESASHIELDSPARKER.COM/GIFT/
12 BEAUTIFUL 4-COLOR CARDS

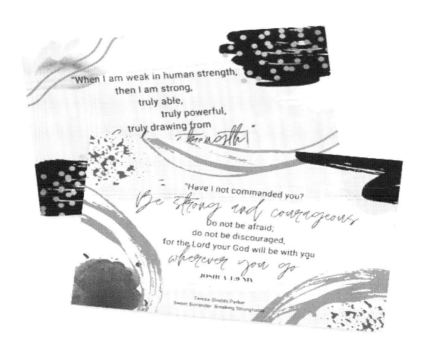

NEXT STEPS

"When I am weak in human strength,
then I am strong, truly able,
truly powerful,
truly drawing from God's strength."

2 COR 12:10 AMP

Made in the USA
Columbia, SC
25 August 2021